Understanding Wellbeing

An Introduction for Students and Practitioners
of Healt'

Health and Social Care titles available from Lantern Publishing Ltd

Clinical Skills for Student Nurses edited by Robin Richardson
ISBN 978 1 906052 04 1
Understanding Research and Evidence-based Practice by Bruce Lindsay
ISBN 978 1 906052 01 0
Values for Care Practice by Sue Cuthbert and Jan Quallington
ISBN 978 1 906052 05 8
Communication and Interpersonal Skills by Elaine Donnelly and
  Lindsey Neville
ISBN 978 1 906052 06 5
Numeracy, Clinical Calculations and Basic Statistics by Neil Davison
ISBN 978 1 906052 07 2
Essential Study Skills edited by Marjorie Lloyd and Peggy Murphy
ISBN 978 1 906052 14 0
Safe and Clean Care by Tina Tilmouth with Simon Tilmouth
ISBN 978 1 906052 08 9
Neonatal Care edited by Amanda Williamson and Kenda Crozier
ISBN 978 1 906052 09 6
Fundamentals of Diagnostic Imaging edited by Anne-Marie Dixon
ISBN 978 1 906052 10 2
Fundamentals of Nursing Care by Anne Llewellyn and Sally Hayes
ISBN 978 1 906052 13 3
The Care and Wellbeing of Older People edited by Angela Kydd, Tim Duffy
  and F.J. Raymond Duffy
ISBN 978 1 906052 15 7
Palliative Care edited by Elaine Stevens and Janette Edwards
ISBN 978 1 906052 16 4
Nursing in the UK: A Handbook for Nurses from Overseas
by Wendy Benbow and Gill Jordan
ISBN 978 1 906052 00 3
Interpersonal Skills for the People Professions edited by Lindsey Neville
ISBN 978 1 906052 18 8
Understanding and Helping People in Crisis by Elaine Donnelly, Briony Williams
  and Tess Parkinson
ISBN 978 1 906052 21 8
A Handbook for Student Nurses by Wendy Benbow and Gill Jordan
ISBN 978 1 906052 19 5
Professional Practice in Public Health edited by Jill Stewart and Yvonne Cornish
ISBN 978 1 906052 20 1

Understanding Wellbeing

An Introduction for Students and Practitioners
of Health and Social Care

Edited by Anneyce Knight and Allan McNaught

Lantern

ISBN: 978 1 908625 00 7
First published in 2011 by Lantern Publishing Limited

Lantern Publishing Limited, The Old Hayloft, Vantage Business Park,
Bloxham Road, Banbury, OX16 9UX
www.lanternpublishing.co.uk

British Library Cataloguing in Publication Data
A catalogue record for this book is available from the British Library

The authors and publisher have made every attempt to ensure the content of this book is up
to date and accurate. However, healthcare knowledge and information is changing all the time
so the reader is advised to double-check any information in this text on drug usage, treatment
procedures, the use of equipment, etc. to confirm that it complies with the latest safety
recommendations, standards of practice and legislation, as well as local Trust policies and
procedures. Students are advised to check with their tutor and/or mentor before carrying
out any of the procedures in this textbook.

Production project management by Deer Park Productions
Typeset by Kestrel Data, Exeter, Devon
Cover design by Andrew Magee Design Ltd
Printed and bound by the MPG Books Group Ltd, UK
Distributed by NBN International, 10 Thornbury Road, Plymouth, PL6 7PP, UK

This book is dedicated to our children, friends, families and colleagues.

Contents

Part 3: Physical Aspects of Wellbeing

Part 4: Social Approaches to Wellbeing

List of Abbreviations and Acronyms

5-HT	Serotonin
5-HTT (SERT)	Serotonin Re-uptake Transporter
ABC	Affective, Behavioural, Cognitive
ACTH	Adrenocorticotropic Hormone
ADHD	Attention Deficit Hyperactivity Disorder
ADL	Activities of Daily Living
A&E	Accident and Emergency
ALSPAC	Avon Longitudinal Study of Parents and Children
AMOSSHE	Association of Managers of Student Services In Higher Education
BBC	British Broadcasting Corporation
BDI	Beck Depression Inventory
BDNF	Brain-derived Neurotropic Factor
BET	Behaviour, Emotions, Thinking
BMI	Body Mass Index
BTCV	British Trust for Conservation Volunteers
CABE	Commission for Architecture and the Built Environment
CBT	Cognitive Behavioural Therapy
CDC	US Centers for Diseases Control
CFS	Chronic Fatigue Syndrome
CHF	Congestive Heart Failure
CNVs	Copy Number Variants
DCLG	Department for Communities and Local Government
DCSF	Department for Children, Schools and Families
DEFRA	Department for Environment, Food and Rural Affairs
DH	Department of Health
DWP	Department for Work and Pensions
ECM	Every Child Matters
ESRC	Economic and Social Research Council
FSA	Food Standards Agency
FTO	Fused Toes and Other abnormalities (gene)
GDP	Gross Domestic Product
GHI	Gross Happiness Index
GNP	Gross National Product
GP	General Practitioner
HAM-D	Hamilton Rating Scale for Depression

HDI	Human Development Index
HEFCE	Higher Education Funding Council for England
HEI	Higher Education Institutions
HHSRS	Housing Health and Safety Rating System
HImP	Health Improvement Plan
HIV	Human Immunodeficiency Virus
HM	Her Majesty
HPA	Hypothalamic-pituitary-adrenal
HRQL	Health-related Quality of Life
HSE	Heath and Safety Executive
IBD	Irritable Bowel Disease
IDRC	International Development Research Centre
JASP	Joint Approach to Social Policy
JIP	Joint Investment Plan
JSNA	Joint Strategic Needs Assessment
LA	Local Authority
LAA	Local Area Agreement
LDL	Low-density Lipoprotein
LSP	Local Strategic Partnerships
MAA	Multi-Area Agreements
MBCT	Mindfulness-based Cognitive Therapy
MDD	Major Depressive Disorder
MHC	Major Histocompatibility Complex
MMR	Measles, Mumps and Rubella vaccine
MOH	Ministry of Health
MP	Member of Parliament
mRNAs	Messenger Ribonucleic Acids
NCB	National Children's Bureau
NCLSCS	National College for Leadership of Schools and Children's Services
NEF	New Economics Foundation
NHS	National Health Service
NICE	National Institute for Health and Clinical Excellence
NK	Natural Killer
nREM	non Rapid Eye Movement
ODPM	Office of Deputy Prime Minister
OECD	Organisation for Economic Cooperation and Development
OFSTED	Office for Standards in Education
ONS	Office for National Statistics
PCS	Physical Component Scores
PCT	Primary Care Trust
PEST	Political, Economic, Socio-cultural and Technological
PISA	Programme for International Student Assessment
PNI	Psychoneuroimmunology
POMS	Positive and negative effect and mood state in specific interventions
PSA	Public Service Agreements
PSHE	Personal, Social, Health and Economic education

PWB	Psychological Wellbeing (Ryff's Scales)
QoL	Quality of Life
RCP	Royal College of Psychiatrists
REM	Rapid Eye Movement (sleeping)
RENU	Renewable Utilities Nottinghamshire
SAD	Seasonal Affective Disorder
SARS	Severe Acute Respiratory Syndrome
SEAL	Social and Emotional Aspects of Learning
SERT (5-HTT)	Serotonin Re-uptake Transporter
SEU	Social Exclusion Unit
SSRI	Serotonin-selective Re-uptake Inhibitor
STD	Sexually Transmitted Disease
SWB	Subjective Wellbeing
SWS	Slow Wave Sleep
TNF-α	Tumour Necrosing Factor
TPB	Theory of Planned Behaviour
TPH2	Tryptophan Hydroxylase-2 gene
TRA	Theory of Reasoned Action
TSO	The Stationery Office
UK	United Kingdom
UN	United Nations
UNDP	United Nations Development Programme
UNICEF	United Nations Children's Fund (formerly United Nations International Children's Emergency Fund)
US	United States
USA	United States of America
USHA	University Safety and Health Association
VE	Virtue Ethics
WBT	Wellbeing Therapy
WHO	World Health Organization

The Contributors

Alfonso Jimenez PhD, BSc, CSCS*D, NSCA-CPT*D

Alfonso Jimenez is Professor of Sports Sciences and Head of the Centre for Sports Sciences and Human Performance at the University of Greenwich. He holds a PhD in Physiology, a Bachelor degree in Exercise Sciences, and different professional accreditations and certifications as CSCS and NSCA-CPT (both Recertified with Distinction). In 2007 he completed a postdoctoral training at Arizona State University (Exercise and Wellness Department). Professor Jimenez serves as Chairman of the Standards Council at the European Health and Fitness Association (**www.ehfa.eu**), a not-for-profit association based in Brussels that currently represents approximately 9000 health clubs and leisure centres and 18 national associations spread across 22 European countries. The EHFA Standards Council is the independent body able to provide strategic advice, guidance and direction to EHFA, in relation to standards, to achieve the EHFA's main goal to get more people more active, more often. In this role Professor Jimenez is leading different groups of experts from all of Europe to establish the Standards about people (regarding the European Qualifications Framework), programmes (evidence-based structured exercise interventions) and places (sports facilities) at European level. He is serving as consultant for different projects, companies and institutions, including regional governments and health care providers.

Allan McNaught PhD, MPhil, BSc (Hons), FRSM

Allan McNaught has worked in health care management, health reform and management strengthening in the UK, Africa, Russia and the former USSR, Bosnia, Serbia and the FYR, as well as in Central and South America and the Caribbean. His work has mainly focused on health system improvement through modernisation and strategic planning of hospital services, together with developing primary care systems and developing local capacity through the establishment of university programmes in health policy, health planning and management. Allan is head of the Social Work and Health Development Department of the University of Greenwich. His main academic interest is in inter-ethnic differences in health care.

Anne Gill SRN, DipN (Lond), Cert Ed, BSc (Hons), MSc

Anne Gill has a nursing background and has worked in Australia, Germany, Scotland and England. She has been involved in continuing professional development for health and social care workers since 1984. A more recent but related interest is in flexible learning for mature students utilising e.learning and blended learning. She is currently programme leader for a Foundation Degree in Care Management involving e.learning plus flexible attendance. She was also part of a team that developed a programme of clinical supervisions workshops that is being used by NHS trusts throughout South-East England. Anne is currently a Senior Lecturer at the University of Greenwich.

Anneyce Knight MSc, PGCE, BA (Hons), RN

Anneyce Knight worked within the NHS and the private sector in a number of roles before taking up her current position as Senior Lecturer in the University of Greenwich's School of Health and Social Care. She is programme leader for BSc Health and Combined Studies and has led on the development of a new BSc Health and Wellbeing programme. Her main research interests relate to inequalities in health and social inclusion, and wellbeing, and she lectures on health policy and contemporary health and wellbeing issues at undergraduate and postgraduate level, both at the University and internationally. She is also European Lead for the School and has presented papers nationally and internationally.

Benjamin (Ben) M.S. Bruneau BA (Hons), MSc, PhD, MInstM, RN, DN, RMN, NDNC, PWT, PGCE, PGCEA, FHEA, Chartered Psychologist

Ben Bruneau works as a Senior Lecturer in the Health Development Department of the School of Health and Social Care of the University of Greenwich, London. He is the programme leader for the BSc Honours Complementary Therapies programmes. Prior to moving to this position, he worked as programme leader for the BSc Honours Health programme, Assistant Director of Research for the School, and, for a number of years, as a teacher of nurses in a primary health care setting. He has long researched in the field of personality and, for the last few years, he has focused on the influence of personality on stress. He teaches health psychology and research methods and his teaching and research activities have increased his interest in research approaches and new technologies that facilitate methods of studying relationships among psychological constructs. He is at present particularly involved in research using structural and econometric modelling. His publications include the assessment of stress interventions, the skills and knowledge utilised by health practitioners, and the use of psychometric instruments in the assessment of personality.

Bill Goddard BEd, MEd, MPhil, FRSA, FHEA

Bill Goddard is Principal Lecturer in Education in the School of Education at the University of Greenwich. He has been Director of CPD, Head of the Department of Education Leadership and Development, and Head of the Department of Professional Learning and Development in the School of Education and Training. He is currently programme leader on the Professional Doctorate in Education programme, and was previously the programme leader for the MA in Education and for the BEd (Hons) four-year programme for secondary teacher training.

He has been an external examiner in three British universities and is an ex-CNAA adviser. He has been active in several European research and development projects since 1991, and has taught Masters programmes in The Netherlands and Sweden since 1991. He is currently a Director and Trustee of the Southern Education Leadership Trust (SELT), a charitable company that delivers national leadership training programmes for school leaders and aspiring school leaders in the South of England. A past President of the International Professional Development Association (IPDA), he is Vice-President of The Learning Teacher Network, a European network of teachers engaged in the identification of the future learning needs of teachers, and is the editor of *The Learning Teacher Journal*, a peer-reviewed European journal.

Carlos J. Moreno-Leguizamon BA, MA, PhD

Carlos Moreno-Leguizamon has a social sciences background – medical anthropology and health communication – and has worked in Colombia, the USA, India, Ghana, Tanzania, Kenya and the UK. Professionally, he combines two key areas of experience: on the one hand, programme design, implementation and evaluation of health, cultural and environmental projects from the grass-roots level to the macro institutional level and, on the other, the teaching and researching of health, culture and medical systems. In particular, his research has related to the discourse analysis of illegal drug use, development and environment issues and, above all, health-illness in three medical traditions – Ayurveda, biomedicine and indigenous medicine from Colombia. Currently, as Senior Lecturer and programme leader for MSc Research at the School of Health and Social Care at the University of Greenwich, he is involved in the implementation of action research projects on black minority and ethnic health issues in South-East England, as well as in the teaching of culture competency and equality and diversity issues to health and social care students.

Christine G. Stacey BSc (Hons), PGDipHE, MA, RN, DNCert, FNP

Christine Stacey has a nursing background and she worked in a variety of clinical settings in the UK before spending 16 years in the developing world where she circumnavigated the globe working with an aid organisation. Her working interest in other health systems led to the University of Greenwich and she was, until recently, the programme leader for Complementary Therapies. Her teaching interests lie with the emerging discipline of Psychoneuroimmunology and the socioeconomic perspectives of health in both traditional environments and via e.learning. Her research interest is with the education and training of student nurses in primary care.

Clarence Spigner MPH, DrPH (USA)

Clarence Spigner's background is medical sociology, anthropology and public health. While a pre-doctoral fellow, he worked as a health planner for the NHS in 1982. He wrote his doctoral dissertation on race, ethnicity and health in the UK and the USA. His area of expertise in the health of the public encompasses race and ethnic relations, health promotion, programme evaluation and health planning. His publications include books on knowledge and perceptions about organ donation and transplantation, tobacco-related behaviour, the intersection of popular culture on perceptions and behaviour, and the African diaspora. He has a visiting professor appointment at the University of Greenwich and is currently professor of Public Health at the University of Washington.

Fiona Bushell BSc (Hons), MSc, PhD, FRSPH

After obtaining a degree in Microbiology, Fiona Bushell retrained as an environmental health officer and worked for three Kent councils. While studying for her MSc in Environmental Health at Thames Polytechnic (now the University of Greenwich), she joined the University of Greenwich as a senior lecturer specialising in food safety and health promotion. She was a lecturer on the BSc Environmental Health programme for 13 years and was programme leader for four years. Her PhD thesis, undertaken with the University of Bradford, examined the adequacy of the education and training of environmental health officers in food control. For the last seven years she has been a senior lecturer in Health Promotion and Public Health at Canterbury Christ Church University teaching undergraduate and postgraduate students. She is currently Pathway Leader of the MSc in Health Promotion and Public Health. Her publications include professional papers and contributions to two books on public health.

Harry Chummun PhD, BSc (Hons), RT, RN

Harry Chummun qualified as an adult nurse in 1976 and worked as charge nurse in various medical wards until 1983. He qualified as a nurse tutor in 1984 and worked in the Middle East as a lecturer practitioner. He returned to England in 1991 and has since worked as a nurse tutor at the University of Greenwich. He obtained his Bachelor degree in Applied Biological Sciences in 1996 and his PhD in Physiology in 2000 from the University of Greenwich. Since 2001, he has been responsible for the implementation of 'genetics and genomics' in the pre-registration programmes for nurses and midwives and in 2010 he was appointed as the Genetics and Genomics Coordinator, pre-registration programme at the University of Greenwich. He has published extensively in professional journals on anatomy and physiology and nursing topics, and continues to contribute chapters in various books. He is also an Associate Lecturer for the Open University and a teaching member of a private company providing education and training for qualified midwives and complementary therapists.

Jill Stewart BSc (Hons), MSc, PhD, PGCE (PCET), MCIEH, FRSPH, FRGS, ACIH

Jill Stewart's environmental health and housing career started in local government, leading to her current post as Senior Lecturer and Research Lead in the Social Work and Health Development Department, School of Health and Social Care, at the University of Greenwich. She currently teaches across public health and housing programmes to postgraduate level and to visiting overseas students. Her main research interests include evidence-based practice and the effectiveness of front-line strategies and interventions in sometimes very challenging public health and housing situations. She pioneered the idea and development of the Chartered Institute of Environmental Health's Private Sector Housing Evidence Base, an online resource available to members, and she was its first editor. Her publications include books and numerous papers published in peer-reviewed and professional journals and she has presented to a range of local, national and international conferences. She is the Public Health Route Leader for the MA Professional Practice in Health and Social Care at the University of Greenwich.

Mark Goss-Sampson MIBiol, PGDip, PhD

Mark Goss-Sampson is a Principal Lecturer in the Centre for Sports Sciences and Human Performance at the University of Greenwich. For the past 15 years he has been teaching in the field of sport, exercise and fitness at both undergraduate and postgraduate levels. He holds a PhD in Neurophysiology and completed his postdoctoral training at the Institute of Child Health, University College London. His first degree was in Biochemistry and Physiology from the University of London. His principal research is in the analysis of human movement and sensorimotor coordination ranging across sports performance, work-based ergonomics and the effects of training programmes on activities of daily living and wellbeing in the elderly population. He has also served as a consultant for projects relating to the health care industry and government bodies.

Nevin Mehmet BSc (Hons), PGDipHE

Nevin Mehmet's career in health started within complementary medicine, leading to her current post as a Senior Lecturer in the Social Work and Health Development Department, School of Health and Social Care at the University of Greenwich. During her academic development she has had a growing and active interest in ethics and ethical decision making within health care. She currently teaches ethics across a range of programmes including public health, health, social work and nursing. Her main research interests lie in the area of values and decision making and she is currently completing her MA in Medical Ethics and Law at Keele University.

Kate Beaven-Marks MSc, CMIOSH, MIRM, MinstLM, PDHyp, BCH, CI

Kate Beaven-Marks is the Occupational Health and Safety Assistant Manager with the University of East London. She has a wealth of knowledge in occupational health and health and safety gained from a career that has ranged from heavy industry through to higher education. Recently she has developed a range of wellbeing initiatives for staff and students, including the introduction of a stress management awareness training programme and a series of 'WISE UP' campaigns promoting wellbeing and health. She draws on her professional communication skills, qualifications and experience, as well as her skills and experience as a hypnotist, hypnotherapist and teacher in this field. She has lectured and taught both in Europe and internationally on the use of positive and directional language for enhanced communication effectiveness. Her skills, knowledge and experience have combined to create a specific method for teaching professionals how to effectively enhance their communication and presentation skills. Currently she is a student on the EdD programme at the University of Greenwich, and her research focuses on the impact of the National Occupational Standards on hypnotherapy teaching and learning in the UK.

Qaisra E. Khan BA (Hons) MA

Qaisra Khan is an experienced public sector professional who has undertaken a number of roles ranging from local councillor and social services inspector to care coordinator. She has worked as Spiritual and Cultural Care Coordinator at Oxleas NHS Trust since 2004. She has been a visiting lecturer at St Mary's University College, Twickenham for over 10 years and has lectured on the University of Greenwich Dark Empire course for three years. She has recently presented a session on mental health awareness for Muslim Spiritual Care Provision in the NHS, a project of the Muslim Council of Britain. Her education includes an MA in Islamic Cultures and Societies, School of African and Oriental Studies, University of London and a BA (Joint Honours) in History and Archaeology, St David's University College, University of Wales. The BA involved a year's study of Christian theology. Publications include public inspection reports, contributions to the Runnymede Trust journal, *Life in the Day: A Recovery Journal* by Pavillion and *MCT* magazine for multicultural teaching. She has recently received a long service award for being a school governor for over 10 years.

Stella Jones-Devitt BA (Hons), MEd, MSc, Fellow HEA, Teaching Fellow York St John University

Stella Jones-Devitt works at Teesside University and is responsible for overseeing the educational quality of employer engagement provision. Prior to this, she was head of subject for health studies and community engagement at York St John University. She has taken an eclectic educational route with a first degree in graphic design and higher degrees in health-related fitness and health promotion and education. This has been matched by a corresponding occupational route that has resulted in working as a freelance book designer; developing health and wellbeing programmes for organisations and individuals; and lecturing and teaching experience that encompasses everything from basic adult education to the facilitation of Master's level learning. Her current academic interests concern: developing critical thinking approaches in academic practice – specifically in the context of health and social care; knowledge economies and workforce development; the socio-political context of higher education; the feasibility of inter-professional working in an increasingly marketised world; and the values and effectiveness of health-promoting practice and its relevance to the general population.

Simten Malhan PhD

Simten Malhan gained her PhD with her thesis on *The Relationship Between Quality of Life and Health Marketing* from the University of Hacettepe in 2004. From 2002 to 2005 she worked on a Turkish Burden of Disease study as the Director of Intervention Cost, a project that was financed by the World Bank. She became an associate professor in 2008. Also in 2008 she became head of the Medical Document Department in Baskent University. She has authored and co-authored over 100 papers and conference contributions. She has four books published in the field of quality of life and economic evaluation in health care. She teaches on a variety of courses at Baskent University at Ankara in Turkey in the Department of Health Care Management. She is also a consultant on health reimbursement systems in Turkey.

Silvano Zanuso MSc, PhD

Silvano Zanuso received his Bachelor degree in Exercise Science at the University of Padua, his Master of Science at Manchester Metropolitan University and his PhD in Exercise Physiology at the Universidad Europea de Madrid. He is the senior scientific adviser of the Technogym Medical Scientific Department. He is contact professor at the Faculty of Medicine of Padua University in the Department of Exercise Science. His main scientific interest is in the effects of physical activity and exercise on subjects with metabolic disorders. He is consultant for health promotion for different governments and public institutions. He has held conferences and educational programmes in more than 20 countries and currently publishes in scientific indexed journals.

Stuart Spear BA (Hons)

Stuart Spear has worked as a journalist for over 15 years, specialising in food policy, housing, health and safety, environmental protection and public health. For six years he was the editor of *EHP*, the Chartered Institute of Environmental Health's monthly magazine, which goes out to environmental health officers nationally. Before that he was deputy editor of the weekly news magazine *Environmental Health News*. He has written extensively about all aspects of food including food safety, sustainability, nutrition and food production. Since going freelance in early 2010 he has been doing Department of Health funded research into the role local government plays in developing the national wellbeing agenda. He continues to write for a number of publications on food policy and gives talks on wellbeing.

Veronica Habgood BSc, MSc, MCIEH

Following a degree in Environmental Science, Veronica Habgood worked for a number of years as an environmental health officer in Suffolk and London, concurrently undertaking further study in environmental protection. She has worked at the University of Greenwich since 1989, lecturing primarily in environmental protection, public health and the environment–health interface, and she is a contributor to a number of established publications. She is currently the Director of Learning and Quality in the School of Health and Social Care at the University of Greenwich, and a corporate member of the Chartered Institute of Environmental Health.

Introduction

Anneyce Knight and Allan McNaught

WHAT IS WELLBEING?

The perceived limitations of concepts of health have led to notions of 'wellness' and 'wellbeing' emerging as major organising concepts around which to both analyse and to provide services and initiatives to enhance the quality of life of populations, communities, families and individuals. Traditionally, wellbeing is perceived to be a construct that conceptualises health as a state beyond the 'absence of disease' and that incorporates subjective feelings of happiness and contentment with spiritual and socio-economic circumstances. This is reflected, in particular, by the WHO definition of health as 'a state of complete physical, mental and social wellbeing and not merely the absence of disease or infirmity' (WHO, 1946). The WHO subsequently developed this definition within the Ottawa Charter of 1986 to affirm that 'Health is a resource for everyday life, not the object of living. It is a positive concept emphasising social and personal resources as well as physical capabilities' and 'a resource that permits people to lead individually, socially and economically productive lives'. Within this expanded definition is embedded the notion of wellbeing. Contemporary concepts of wellbeing have developed this further by advancing a more holistic, multifactorial and multidisciplinary explanation of what it is to be 'well' in modern society.

This broadened conceptual landscape has provided a rich theoretical space that has energised discussions about public health, and has made more explicit the linkages between the subjective and objective aspects of wellbeing. In so doing, it has engendered greater awareness of the socio-political forces that shape health and wellbeing in society. The contextualisation of biomedical health, which was a by-product of this process, made it obvious to many that action on wellbeing in contemporary society could not appropriately be led by vertical health administration agencies. It was therefore not surprising that local authorities were given authority to exercise 'wellbeing powers' under Section 2 of the Local Government Act 2000. The creation of local strategic partnerships (LSPs) led to greater complexity in our understanding of what constitutes wellbeing, as local authorities sought to deliver a wide range of initiatives under these newly awarded powers.

It is interesting to note that this complexity and confusion is further reflected in the definitions advanced by different government departments. For example, DEFRA states that wellbeing is achieved when

> basic needs are met, that individuals have a sense of purpose, that they feel able to achieve important personal goals and participate in society. It is enhanced by conditions that include supportive personal relationships, strong and inclusive communities, good health, financial and personal security, rewarding employment, and a healthy and attractive environment. (DEFRA, 2009, p. 119)

In contrast, just prior to the General Election in May 2010, the government, in *New Horizons*, stated that wellbeing is 'A positive state of mind and body, feeling safe and able to cope, with a sense of connection with people, communities and the wider environment' (HM Government, 2010, p. 12), with the particular focus on mental wellbeing. The overall conclusion that can be drawn from these definitions is that wellbeing as a concept is seen as encompassing a positive physical, mental and social state, allowing individuals to participate in society and achieve their personal goals. This has been expressed in differing ways in different policy contexts. However, these contextual differences should not distract us from the fact that the same phenomena is being described and that there are shared objectives in its attempted operationalisation.

New Labour launched its *Health, Work and Wellbeing* project in 2005 (www.workingforhealth.gov.uk), putting wellbeing even more firmly on the political agenda. Subsequently, with the publication of the Sustainable Development Strategy *Securing the Future* (DEFRA, 2006), measures were included for wellbeing for the first time. More recently the *NHS Health and Wellbeing Review: Interim Report* (DH, 2009) focused on the health and wellbeing of NHS staff, followed by the publication of the final report on 23 November 2009. This sets out recommendations for improving the provision of health and wellbeing across the NHS. Health and wellbeing is seen as an important contributory factor to delivering high-quality care in the NHS. The report emphasises that health and wellbeing are not only individual considerations, but also issues for organisations as a whole.

The current (2011) coalition government continues to have an agenda for wellbeing. As part of the proposed NHS restructuring, the public health function will be transferred from the NHS to local authorities and new partnerships will be made based on Health and Wellbeing Boards. It has also been stated that wellbeing should inform the policy-making process. With this political agenda in mind, there is potential for partnership working with effective monitoring and evaluation of wellbeing policies and projects and the development of a stronger evidence base. This will be facilitated by the decision to include questions on subjective wellbeing in the next UK national census – an innovation that has already been adopted in a number of other countries.

THE AIMS AND CONTENT OF THIS BOOK

This book aims to further our understanding of wellbeing within contemporary UK society at an individual, family, community and societal level for policy makers, health scientists, health, social care and wellbeing students and practitioners. This book demonstrates the complexity of wellbeing and that wellbeing is relevant irrespective of whether a person is well or has a physical or mental illness or disability. Wellbeing is also a powerful organising concept for framing relevant social policies. These are issues that are being grappled with by a wide spectrum of countries, and this book includes some elements of this broader debate. The multifaceted nature of wellbeing means that creativity, innovation and an unprecedented level of multiagency and professional working will be required if the goal of 'Wellbeing for All' is to be attained. This book seeks to inform this process.

The book is divided into two sections. The first part deals with more conceptual and strategic aspects of wellbeing, including attempting to prove a definitional framework, exploration of the underpinning ethical and philosophical issues, and approaches to monitoring and evaluating wellbeing projects and initiatives. These chapters emphasise our thinking that the pursuit of wellbeing has to be underpinned by something more substantial than good feeling. Projects and initiatives need conceptual, philosophical and ethical clarity. In addition, aims and objectives need to be formulated in such a way that makes them capable of operationalisation and capable of evaluation.

Section two has three foci: the psychological, physical and social aspects of wellbeing. Each chapter seeks to draw together theory, practice and examples within a critical framework to enable students and practitioners to develop a level of mastery of the concept of wellbeing, its various components and an understanding of real-life experiences of wellbeing via case studies, activities and reflection.

This book does not claim to be the last contribution to the topic, but one which attempts to advance the level of debate and discourse, while providing a more contextualised approach to one of the most significant issues in social policy in the modern world.

Part 1: Overview

Chapter 1

Defining Wellbeing

Allan McNaught

Learning outcomes

In this chapter you will learn how to:

- develop working definitions of wellbeing within a framework that will enable you to capture the complexity of the concept;

- compare and contrast the scope and the different components of wellbeing;

- identify the critical connections and interdependencies between the different components of wellbeing.

This chapter seeks to explore wellbeing as a free-standing, multilevelled and complex social construct. The chapter will argue that 'health' is but one component of wellbeing and, while the customary coupling extends 'health' to encompass the emotional and the psychological (and maybe even 'holistic'), it pre-empts our understanding and debates about 'wellbeing'. Wellbeing is a complex, confusing and contested field that would benefit from a framework within which to locate more specific definitions, and to tease out interconnections and cross-cutting issues. The prime objective of this chapter is to give readers of this book a steer by providing a definitional topography for the concept of wellbeing. By providing such a framework, this chapter seeks to make a contribution towards the thinking and discourse about wellbeing, and to assist the reader in locating the individual chapters within a broader context, while also recognising their boundaries/limitations.

INTRODUCTION

Concern with wellbeing has generated a considerable body of literature and research on its many facets and meanings. There is an increasing acceptance that so-called 'objective' measures of social and economic progress are insufficient to analyse and describe human wellbeing, whether at an individual, family, community or societal level. Wellbeing is a feel-good concept that has occupied our 'assumptive world'; it is a concept that is freely used in modern policy discourse, and has become an integral objective in many policy domains, usually without explicit definition. No one seriously opposes this development, although some commentators are amused at the onward march of 'happiness science'. The volume of literature, the elasticity of the concept, and its steady incorporation into the national political and social policy agenda, suggest that the concern and the issues demand serious attention by those concerned with human health and social welfare.

Wellbeing as a concept is frequently coupled with 'health', as in the term 'health and wellbeing'. It will be argued that wellbeing is a broader construct that has a certain moral and philosophical energy: it facilitates reflection on the human condition and provides the backdrop to public policy making and research aimed at the promotion of wellbeing as a desirable state. Therefore, wellbeing is conceptualised as an ideal state of being or existence that we and policy makers strive for, as a contemporary variant of the good life.

Background

The word 'wellbeing' has slipped into our day-to-day discussions, including in 'pop psychology', a range of social policy domains and various fields of academic research. There are competing and contradictory definitions in the literature and some works about wellbeing discuss it extensively, though without actually defining it, or claiming that a definition is impossible. Even when the term is used it is sometimes not clear if it is something profound or just a linguistic flourish. Figure 1.1 shows some of the linguistic issues with the use of the term 'wellbeing'.

Most contemporary discussions of wellbeing start from the WHO definition that 'health is not the mere absence of diseases, but a state of wellbeing' (WHO, 1947). This early coupling has led to a tradition of health being regarded as the province of biomedicine and objectivity, while wellbeing was associated with emotional and psychological states, or subjective wellbeing, and the growth of a specific body of literature concerned with measuring wellbeing as a psychological construct,

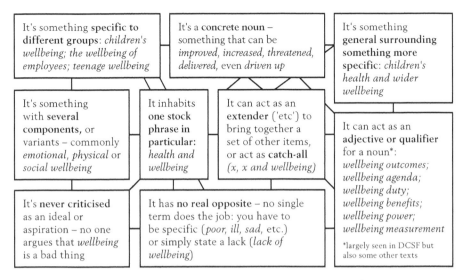

Figure 1.1 The use of the term wellbeing (source: Ereaut and Wright, 2008, reproduced with permission)

as outlined in Chapter 6. The individualisation and internalisation of wellbeing is also expressed in the recent development of positive psychology or 'happiness science'. Interestingly, within the construction of wellbeing as a psychological, subjective phenomenon, some objective elements are usually cited, relating to familial, community and social factors, the built environment and the individual's command over or access to resources. That being said, subjective wellbeing is important in that it tries to encapsulate a notion of how people cope, thrive and survive, individually and collectively.

However, wellbeing can be assessed as both an objective and subjective construct. Because of the complexity of the concept, wellbeing measurement must recognise its multifactorial nature and the need for a range of tools and disciplines, as well as social and policy changes, to be involved in its promotion, measurement and expression. Clearly, some of these instruments will be less validated than others, but this should not detract from the overall integrity of the concept and the approach. For example, an assessment of how well or happy people feel, as individuals or as societies, has been demonstrated by the psychological wellbeing literature (see Chapter 6). Diener and Seligman (2004) have argued that social policy formulation should take subjective wellbeing into account, and should also attempt to monitor it on a longitudinal basis to inform policy. Subjective wellbeing has also been taken up by economists, and transformed into the 'Quality of Life' concept. Quality of life usually refers to the degree to which a person's life is desirable versus undesirable, often with an emphasis on external components such as environmental factors and income. In contrast to subjective wellbeing, which is based on inner/psychological experiences, quality of life is often expressed as more 'objective' and describes the circumstances of a person's life rather than his or her reaction to those circumstances.

Clearly, the quality of life concept brings another dimension to our consideration of wellbeing, and illustrates the obvious shortcoming of subjective wellbeing. By so doing, it makes the point that it might be more realistic to view wellbeing as a field of study that encompasses a range of specialist areas of research and practice aimed at understanding and promoting a positive state of existence in specific domains and for specific populations or socio-economic and political entities. We are only able to make sense of the varied literature and competing definitions by taking a broader approach that contextualises and incorporates operational definitions, such as happiness, quality of life, and objective and subjective wellbeing. Because of this complexity, the search for a generally accepted definition of wellbeing is fruitless, frustrating and ultimately impossible.

These concepts have also been extended to the societal level, with the King of Bhutan suggesting the development of a Gross Happiness Index (GHI) to replace Gross National Product (GNP) as an index of national wellbeing. President Sarkozy of France has been the first developed-country politician to formally adopt this approach, with the commissioning of a group led by the economist Joseph Stiglitz to develop happiness measures for France. Also, according to Stratton (2010), 'The UK government is poised to start measuring people's psychological and environmental wellbeing, bidding to be among the first countries to officially monitor happiness.' Concepts and definitions of wellbeing can therefore be perceived to be wrapped around the whole structure of humanity and its social and ecological existence. The next section will attempt to outline a 'definitional framework for the concept of wellbeing'. This will provide a framework for more specific definitions and provide an overall framework for understanding the concept of wellbeing.

AN OVERVIEW OF THE FIELD OF STUDY

For Felce and Perry (1995), wellbeing '… comprises objective descriptors and subjective evaluations of physical, material, social and emotional wellbeing, together with the extent of personal development and purposeful activity, all weighted by a personal set of values' (Felce and Perry, 1995, p. 60). For Bentham (1817) 'Directly or indirectly, wellbeing, in some shape or other ... is the subject of every thought, and object of every action, on the part of every known Being ... nor can any intelligible reason be given for desiring that it should be otherwise' (Bentham, 1817, p. 79).

Figure 1.2 shows what I term a definitional framework for the concept of wellbeing. At this level, wellbeing is a macro concept or an area of study concerned with the objective and subjective assessment of how human beings survive, thrive and function.

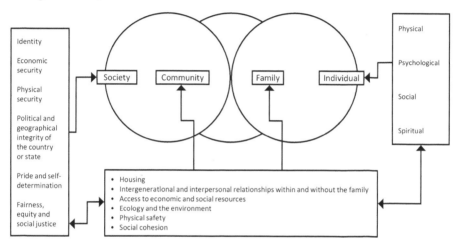

Figure 1.2 A structured framework for defining wellbeing (Dr Allan McNaught, October 2010)

The importance of this framework is that it extends the definition and concept of wellbeing to a range of different dimensions beyond individual subjectivity, and removes the conventional linking with 'health' to include the family, community and society as a whole. It also repositions and broadens the factors identified with individual wellbeing.

This model presents wellbeing as a dynamic process that gives people a sense of how their lives are going, through the interaction between their circumstances, activities and psychological resources, and includes their interpersonal interactions with significant social formations (the family and their community) within society. It is important that individuals, families and communities are not conceptualised as passive actors to whom others deliver wellbeing as a product. Wellbeing is also a result of their own actions and their own social and political preferences and interventions to change their circumstances and to influence the governance of their society to support what they perceive to be 'good'.

As a result of this dynamism, high levels of wellbeing and consciousness about what wellbeing might mean give the motivation and capacity to respond to difficult circumstances, to innovate, challenge and constructively engage with other people and the world around us. As well as representing a highly effective way of bringing about good outcomes in many different areas our lives, there is also a strong case for regarding wellbeing as an ultimate goal of human endeavour, as indicated by Bentham's quote above.

Individual wellbeing

This area has been the focus of much of the theorising and research on wellbeing. Diener (2005), particularly, has researched and written extensively on all aspects of wellbeing. He has defined subjective wellbeing as

> all of the various types of evaluations, both positive and negative, that people make of their lives. It includes reflective cognitive evaluations, such as life satisfaction and work satisfaction, interest and engagement, and affective reactions to life events, such as joy and sadness. Thus, subjective wellbeing is an umbrella term for the different valuations people make regarding their lives, the events happening to them, their bodies and minds, and the circumstances in which they live. (Diener, p. 2)

Individual wellbeing, by its nature, is a multidimensional concept and there has been a multitude of definitions as to what it might mean. Within the literature there is a variation between those who are predisposed to the measurement of attitudes or attributes, and those who link these subjective feelings with certain defined social situations. Robinson (2010), for example, identified the following five categories of wellbeing as essential to everyone:

- **career wellbeing**: how you occupy your time – or simply liking what you do every day;
- **social wellbeing**: having strong relationships and love in your life;
- **financial wellbeing**: effectively managing your economic life;
- **physical wellbeing**: having good health and enough energy to get things done on a daily basis;
- **community wellbeing**: the sense of engagement you have with the area where you live.

It is notable that Robinson's taxonomy does not explicitly mention the family, although this can, by inference, be included in 'social wellbeing', while 'community wellbeing' is perceived purely in terms of relationships. These varying concepts of wellbeing have been augmented by studies of happiness; and happiness has been posited as the ultimate form of individual wellbeing.

Activity 1.1 Reflective exercise

Robinson identified five components of individual wellbeing. Rank these components in the order that reflects their importance to your individual wellbeing.

1. How would you explain your order of preference?
2. How would you feel if your ranking were completely reversed? Can you explain your feelings about this reordering?

In Figure 1.2, individual wellbeing is shown to be influenced by a combination of physical, psychological, spiritual/moral and social factors. Most instruments that attempt to measure individual wellbeing or quality of life try to capture the impact of these factors on the individual's subjective experience (internal world). The framework also suggests that individual wellbeing is conditioned by the nature of the context in which the individual is situated and can only be understood within that context.

Family wellbeing

Paraphrasing Diener (2005), family wellbeing refers to all of the various types of evaluations, both positive and negative, that a family make of their lives. It includes reflective cognitive evaluations, such as life satisfaction and work satisfaction, interest and engagement, the quality of interpersonal and intergenerational relationships, family access to economic and other resources, and the overall circumstances in which they live (Diener, 2005, p. 2).

Individual and family wellbeing are strongly related; most individuals live within the context of a family (however defined), and the quality of personal relationships and the access to physical and other resources are generally a feature of personal and family wellbeing. These resources are many and varied – child care, caring for the disabled, pooling resources for day-to-day living, providing or facilitating economic opportunities for family members – and these are all part of the resources that promote wellbeing.

Concern with family functioning and family wellbeing has been an enduring feature of social policy, but what does this actually mean? Wollny *et al.* (2010) have undertaken an extensive review of the literature. They argue that the available literature approaches the understanding and measurement of family wellbeing through the prism of varying frameworks based on:

- ecological systems theory;
- resource theory;
- family systems theory.

Ecological systems theory

Ecology is the study of the representation of living organisms and the interactions among and between organisms and their environments. In human ecological systems theory the wellbeing of humans is embedded within the wellbeing of their biological, physical and social environments, in other words: 'the wellbeing of individuals and families cannot be considered apart from the wellbeing of the whole ecosystem' (Rettig and Leichtentritt, 1999, p. 309). When applied to families, it is argued that their wellbeing and environments are linked through interactions and interdependent relationships. For example, an ecological perspective is now standard in the context of family interventions and programmes (Barnes *et al.*, 2005).

Voydanoff (2007) also identifies six categories of family, work and community characteristics derived from an analysis of empirical research:

- structure;
- social organisation;
- norms and collective efficacy;
- support (the provision or receipt of instrumental or emotional social support);
- orientations (the salience, commitment, involvement, aspirations);
- quality (subjective evaluation of multidimensional domains).

Together, the ecological levels and categories serve as a framework for examining links between family, work and community.

Resource theory

Resource theory provides researchers with a way of conceptualising the interpersonal 'resource exchanges' in family relationships. To do this it identifies six interdependent classes of resource:

- love;
- services;
- goods;
- money;
- information;
- status.

Resource theory thus defines family wellbeing as a multidimensional concept. It uses the six classes of resource to guide the definition of the content of family life, from which follows the development of measures and interpretation of findings. It also links together the concept of 'personal needs' being met through 'resources' that in turn produce 'life satisfactions'. Further arguments for the theory's relevance to family wellbeing research are its recognition of the importance of both economic and social-psychological human needs and that it explicitly acknowledges the interaction between these domains.

Family systems theory

These theories view a family as an organised hierarchy of subsystems, including individuals, subsets of individuals and the overall combination of family members (Bonomi *et al.*, 2005, p. 1128). Psychological or psychosocial family systems theory approaches to understanding the wellbeing of whole families emphasise the organisational complexity of families, their interdependent relationships, interactive patterns and dynamics. In these approaches, whether a family system is 'well' or not is determined by the elements of its internal functioning. The approaches documented in psychological literature on family functioning can be broadly divided according to their focus:

- on the family as an entity – its adjustment and preservation;
- on child development, viewing the family in terms of its contributions to child welfare;
- on the family as a system with internal dynamics that produce developmental and welfare outcomes for its members.

The functioning frameworks that have been described by researchers include elements that are internal to the family as well as family functioning elements that play out externally. The Australian Bureau of Statistics (2002) has developed a family wellbeing model that suggests that family wellbeing is built upon the 'personal resources' of family members and is produced through interactions between 'Family Structures, Family Transitions and Family Functioning', through transactions with individual and societal wellbeing (see also Trewin, 2001).

Community wellbeing

There is no accepted, universally used definition of 'community wellbeing' or a definitive set of community wellbeing indicators in use. However, community wellbeing can be defined as a concept meant to recognise the social, cultural and psychological needs of people, their family, institutions and communities. This definition clearly extends beyond subjective wellbeing and implies consideration of health, poverty, transportation and economic activity, environmental and ecological factors. Kusel (1996) reflected on concerns as to how a community might heal itself to meet the needs of its residents. This ability is conceptualised as 'community capacity' composed of the following components:

- physical capital;
- human capital;
- social capital.

Community capacity was identified as an important factor influencing community wellbeing, while Doak and Kusel (1996) define wellbeing as a function of both socio-economic skills and community capacity. Their work shows that communities with a high socio-economic status do not necessarily have a high community capacity.

Communities can be defined in many ways, and individuals and families can belong to many overlapping and distinctive communities at the same time. Identification with communities is a source of social, psychological, spiritual/moral and physical wellbeing to individuals and families. The wellbeing of particular communities could be adversely affected by external sources and events that can undermine their economic viability, physical security or psychological wellbeing to an extent that the community concerned will find it difficult to experience a high level of wellbeing or, in extremes, to survive.

'Community' has been found to be an influential factor in the success of an intervention, even for interventions purely on the family level, such as parenting classes. These community influences are thought to come about via:

- institutional resources (the quality, quantity and diversity of the learning, recreational, social, educational and health resources of a community);
- relationships and community ties;
- norms and collective efficacy.

Activity 1.2

The City of Happiton Community Wellbeing Plan 2006–2011 has the objective of galvanising the council, the community and other partners to understand and to collaborate on identifying the community wellbeing issues in Happiton, and to agree actions to be taken for improvement. Developed in partnership with the community and key stakeholders, the Community Wellbeing Plan has a vision, goal and seven key objectives:

1. a strong, cohesive and connected community;
2. a safe community;
3. a socially inclusive community;
4. a liveable environment;
5. a healthy community;
6. a community engaged in lifelong learning and employment;
7. a sustainable local economy with a vibrant mix of commercial and social enterprise.

List three policies or activities that would be appropriate for each of these objectives.

Societal wellbeing

The promotion of wellbeing at a societal level is one of the great political, social and economic challenges of our time. Many governments and inter-governmental organisations are now focused on its measurement and enhancement. 'GDP has increasingly become used as a measure of societal wellbeing and changes in the structure of the economy and our society have made it an increasingly poor one' (Stiglitz, 2002). He recommends including other factors, such as sustainability and education. Others have also long recognised that GDP is an inadequate measure to assess societal wellbeing, and there have been numerous suggestions of what else to count to make it a more reliable yardstick. De Leon and Boris (2010) recommended the inclusion of the following estimates in GDP:

1. unpaid and paid care work;
2. levels of child poverty and deprivation;
3. impact of discrimination against social minorities;
4. impact of gender disparities.

Societal wellbeing has been defined as:

> A positive, social and mental state; it is not just the absence of pain, discomfort and incapacity. It arises not only from the action of individuals, but from a host of collective goods and relationships with other people. It requires that basic needs are met, that individuals have a sense of purpose, and that they feel able to achieve important personal goals and participate in society. It is enhanced by conditions that include supportive personal relationships, involvement in empowered communities, good health, financial security, rewarding employment and a healthy and attractive environment. (Skilton, 2009, p. 9)

Skilton disaggregates wellbeing into the following components:

- involvement in empowered communities;
- supportive personal relationships;
- good health;
- financial security;
- rewarding employment; and a
- healthy and attractive environment.

Skilton identifies nine UK wellbeing indices, from a range of sources, as well as 19 datasets that measure aspects of wellbeing, ranging from the *Health Survey for England* through the *British Crime Survey* to the *British Social Attitudes Survey*. We can get a better feel of this document's approach by looking at one area, 'Involvement in empowered communities', that it defines as

> An empowered community can primarily be based on the level of self sufficiency, which may then lead to a greater sense of control over life. Self sufficiency allows people to lead independent lives without the need to require any outside aid, support, or interaction, for survival. This includes having access to key services. (Skilton, 2009, p. 9)

The report then analyses the perceived difficulty of people in the community in accessing key services between 1997/8 and 2006/7. These key services were defined as 'corner shop/supermarket, post office, doctor/hospital'. The report showed that non-car owners experience significant and constant disadvantage compared with car owners. Throughout the report, there are similar attempts to determine how societal wellbeing should and could be measured.

An example of national accounts of wellbeing for the UK was published by the New Economics Foundation (2009). Their 'Framework for National Accounts of Wellbeing' is based on capturing the following:

- Understanding subjective wellbeing as a multifaceted, dynamic combination of different factors has important implications for the way in which it is measured. This requires indicators which look beyond single-item questions and capture more than simply life satisfaction.
- Personal and social dimensions. Measurement of the social dimension of wellbeing (in terms of individuals' subjective reports about how they feel they relate to others).
- Feelings, functioning and psychological resources. Measurement of how well people are doing, in terms of their functioning and the realisation of their potential. Psychological resources, such as resilience, should also be included in any national accounts framework and reflect growing recognition of 'mental capital' as a key component of wellbeing.

Application of the New Economics Foundation's National Accounts of Wellbeing reveals:

- Countries with high levels of personal wellbeing do not necessarily have high levels of social wellbeing, and vice versa. Denmark and Ukraine display unusual stability in coming at the very top and very bottom, respectively, of rankings based on both personal and social wellbeing scores.
- Scandinavian countries are the top performers on overall wellbeing, while Central and Eastern European countries have the lowest wellbeing.
- Despite its relative economic success at the time the survey data were collected, this summary measure nevertheless reveals the UK's distinctly middling performance on wellbeing overall.
- Levels of wellbeing inequality vary considerably between nations.
- Within the UK, clear differences emerged in the character of people's wellbeing between population groups. The Wellbeing Profiles of the youngest and oldest age groups in the UK reveal some striking differences in their wellbeing composition and levels, with particular disparity for the trust and belonging component, with a very low score for the youngest age group and a high score for the oldest.

This approach to societal wellbeing sees it very much as the result of gradualism and working within the status quo. Other approaches raise more fundamental questions about the balance of resources and the aims and outcomes of social and economic policies. Stiglitz has remarked that:

> While we all speak passionately about the importance of democratic principles, we also recognize that our democracies are imperfect, and that some groups' voices are heard more loudly than others. In the arena of international economic policy, the voices of commercial and financial interests are heard far more loudly than those of labour and consumer interests. As just noted, they have tried to convince others, with remarkable success, that there is no conflict of interests – which means that there are no trade-offs. The consequences speak for themselves: the growing dissatisfaction with the reform policies is partly a consequence of the fact that so many have actually been made worse off. In Mexico, for instance, the incomes of the poorest 30 per cent of the population have actually declined over the past 16 years. All of the income gains (reflected in increases in average GDP per capita) have occurred among the richest 30 per cent, and especially among the richest 10 per cent. According to the Inter-American Development Bank, no country in Latin America for which data on income distribution are available can boast a decline in income inequality during the 1990s. (Stiglitz, 2002, p. 25)

Measuring social capital

In trying to develop ways of measuring social capital and its contribution to societal wellbeing, the Australian National Bureau of Statistics did not define the latter, but saw the purpose of their endeavours as the creation of 'a more just and resilient societal system' (Australian National Bureau of Statistics, 2002, p. 8).

Speaking at 'Wellbeing for all? Achieving wellbeing in an unequal world' (2010), the well-known epidemiologist Professor Richard Wilkinson said that in developed nations the degree of inequality – the size of the difference between the incomes of the rich and the poor – correlates with prevalence of a wide range of social and health problems. This includes life expectancy, which is not related to average incomes, but to income differences. He argued that greater social equality is the most important factor in ensuring people's wellbeing. Societies with a bigger gap between the rich and the poor are bad for everyone in them, including the well-off. While greater equality yields the greatest benefits for the poor, the benefits extend to the majority of the population.

The Human Development Index

The United Nations Development Programme (UNDP) Human Development Index (HDI) is another possible measure of societal wellbeing. The first Human Development Report introduced a new way of measuring development by combining indicators of life expectancy, educational attainment and income into a composite human development index, the HDI. The breakthrough for the HDI was the creation of a single statistic that was to serve as a frame of reference for both social and economic development. The HDI sets a minimum and a maximum for each dimension, called goalposts, and then shows where each country stands in relation to these goalposts, expressed as a value between 0 and 1 (see Figure 1.3).

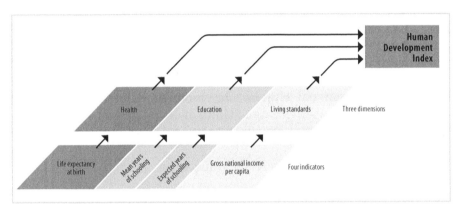

Figure 1.3 Components of the Human Development Index (source: UNDP, 2010, reproduced with permission)

Gross National Happiness

The concept of Gross National Happiness (GNH) was developed in an attempt to define an indicator that measures quality of life or social progress in more holistic and psychological terms than Gross Domestic Product (GDP). The term was coined in 1972 by Bhutan's former King Jigme Singye Wangchuck. He used the phrase to signal his commitment to building an economy that would serve Bhutan's unique culture based on Buddhist spiritual values. At first offered as a casual, offhand remark, the concept was taken seriously and the Centre for Bhutan Studies, under the leadership of Karma Uru, developed a sophisticated survey instrument to measure the population's general level of wellbeing. The Canadian health epidemiologist Michael Pennock had a major role in the design of the instrument, and uses (what he calls) a 'de-Bhutanized' version of the survey in his work in Victoria, British Columbia.

CONCLUSION

This chapter has attempted to provide a definitional framework and an overview of the concept of wellbeing. It has demonstrated that the concept is multilevelled and may be described and measured subjectively and objectively. The achievement of wellbeing, in these terms, is not just a matter of behavioural change or the promotion of 'positive psychology'. Its complexity and its multidimensional nature mean that the pursuit of public policy change and political action is a concomitant of any strategy to change objective reality or circumstances that are assessed as harmful to individual, family, community or societal wellbeing.

Further reading

The United Nations Development Programme (UNDP) and the Human Development Index are available at **http://hdr.undp.org/en/humandev/** The UNDP is concerned with sustainable development and the HDI was created as a way of measuring the range of human and societal capabilities. The annual Human Development Report is one of the cardinal documents on international human development, and is notable for its ranking of societies through the use of the HDI.

New Economics Foundation (NEF) available at **www.neweconomics.org/**
The NEF is an independent think-and-do tank that aims to improve quality of life by promoting innovative solutions that challenge mainstream thinking on economic, environmental and social issues.

Gross National Happiness (GNH). Information about The Centre for Bhutan Studies is available at **www.grossnationalhappiness.com**
The Centre has sponsored the development of policy screening tools that can be used to examine the potential impacts of projects or programmes on GNH.

Chapter 2

Wellbeing and Health

Stella Jones-Devitt

Learning outcomes

In this chapter you will learn how to:

- examine the contested nature of wellbeing in the context of health;

- assess the significance of neo-liberalism to the wellbeing agenda;

- explore ideas concerning how public health practitioners can seek to develop effective practice within this complex ideological climate.

This chapter explores the contested nature of wellbeing and its relationship to health. It starts by presenting a brief history of wellbeing development and then considers contemporary notions of wellbeing within the prevailing UK context. It assesses the ideas and impact of neo-liberalism on everyday life, recognising it as problematic for achieving more holistic notions of wellbeing, especially for those living in social and economic disadvantage. Furthermore, it questions whether public health practice, with its present commitment to achieving wellbeing through social justice, can operate effectively and transparently within a pervasive neo-liberal ideology. Given the rising levels of lifestyle-related conditions and the lack of impact made by existing public health approaches, it is suggested that more direct forms of targeted wellbeing intervention could be explored for the more vulnerable sectors of UK society.

INTRODUCTION

Huppert *et al.* (2008) note that the concept of wellbeing comprises two main elements: feeling good and functioning well. They contend that the feeling good component concerns experiencing happiness, contentment, enjoyment, curiosity and engagement: all are characteristics of those who have positive experiences of their lives. They also contend that the second element, regarding how people function in the world, is equally important for wellbeing. This latter component relates to experiencing positive relationships, having some control over one's life and having a sense of purpose. Positive aspects of wellbeing were being stressed by the end of the 1970s and onwards by Antonovsky (1979) through the theory of 'salutogenesis', which concerned examining why some people remain well while coping successfully with many of life's adverse circumstances. Cronin de Chavez *et al.* (2005) indicate that the concept of salutogenesis is relevant to the critique of wellbeing because it attempts to reverse the measuring of negative health elements (for example, illness and inability to cope) with something of positive valence. While the present climate of neo-liberalism makes some wellbeing approaches less effective, the positive premise offered by salutogenesis forms the basis for further examination of the concept of wellbeing throughout this chapter.

THE CONTESTED NATURE OF WELLBEING

Elements of individual need and the relationship of individuals to the wider world permeate much wellbeing literature and it is difficult to detach the wellbeing agenda from moral connotations. Historically, notions of wellbeing have prevailed since Ancient Greece. Nowakowski (2007) notes that Aristotle proclaimed that a 'good life' is realised through virtuous actions from which human beings attain happiness. According to Ardell (1985; cited in Conrad, 1994), the moral importance of wellbeing was embodied within the Wellness Movement, which encompassed an ideology of both collective and personal moral responsibilities. Conrad suggests that such ideas can be retraced to nineteenth-century American society when widespread anxiety was manifest concerning an apparent lack of national vitality: 'A metaphysical line was forged between health and the vitality of the nation. Physical development was seen as recharging vitality and perhaps more importantly as a step to human perfection' (p. 36). Parallels can also be drawn with the eugenics philosophy that gained strength in Europe and the UK at around the same time.

The moral positioning of wellbeing is not merely a nineteenth-century phenomenon. Fitzgerald (1994) indicates that concepts of wellbeing have continued to broaden, while responsibility for its acquisition has become increasingly diffuse, meaning that a wide array of sources beyond the individual are now deemed accountable. O'Brien (1995) calls this the 'dedifferentiation' of health: 'The extended concept of health-as-wellbeing represents a biological project, requiring knowledge of social, psychological, political and economic processes. It is multifactorial, multisectoral and multidimensional' (p. 196).

Wellbeing appears to be fraught with many contradictory elements. Tesh (1988) identifies that specific tensions occur in the interplay between utilitarian and individualistic values. She notes that a utilitarian approach to wellbeing is advocated for the greater good, while individualistic wellbeing is espoused for the development of autonomy and self-realisation. Seedhouse (1995) asserts that this has led to an unhelpful blurring of wellbeing as a concept, despite many theorists working for over 30 years to determine its meaning: 'while there is some consensus among psychologists that "wellbeing" is constructed out of three components – life satisfaction (which is said to be cognitive), positive affect and negative affect (which are said to be experiences) – beyond this, the nature of "wellbeing" remains mysterious and elusive' (p. 63). This view is confirmed by Cronin de Chavez et al. (2005) who undertook a multidisciplinary literature review of the concept of wellbeing and concluded that – despite the popularity of the notion of wellbeing – it lacks cogency, with little agreement about how it is identified, measured and achieved. Hence, the meaning of 'wellbeing' will depend largely upon the values of those offering the description: wellbeing in some social contexts concerns the ability to freely exchange and convey ideas, while wellbeing in economic terms means having equity of access to material goods and provisions.

Activity 2.1 Defining a concept of wellbeing for health

Consider the contested nature of wellbeing. What constituents do you feel need to be included in a conceptualisation of wellbeing and why? Examine the recent Marmot Review (2010) *Fair Society, Healthy Lives*, available at: *www.marmot-review.org.uk* How does this report propose to enhance wellbeing?

WELLBEING IN THE CONTEXT OF HEALTH

The current political context for wellbeing achievement is problematic within the UK, when removed from discussion of wider social and health inequalities. For example, increasing numbers of people are becoming more obese than ever before at earlier ages, providing epidemiological markers for future lives characterised by chronic disease from puberty onwards. Within the WHO European region, the prevalence of obesity has escalated among all sectors of the population, as indicated in the WHO *Fact Sheet 2.3* (2007) that reports that, within the region, obesity rates across all sectors of the population have tripled since the 1990s. More worryingly, rates among children and adolescents have risen even faster, with a current rate that is ten times higher than during the 1970s. The WHO (2007) report implies that this will create a massive impact on health services as today's overweight children become tomorrow's chronically diseased adults, relying on a lifetime of costly treatments and interventions.

There is considerable evidence that the inequalities gap between the richest and poorest continues to extend. Pickett *et al.* (2005) and latterly Marmot (2010) found that more unequal societies have greater levels of poor health throughout the population, with obesity levels being one obvious and visible marker. The study by Pickett *et al.* linked income inequality in developed countries to obesity, deaths from diabetes and daily calorie intake, and the poorest had the highest levels of obesity allied to the lowest incomes. They argue that policies that promote greater income equality may have effective public health outcomes for overall wellbeing, in addition to wider economic benefits. They contend: 'Because the behaviour changes needed to improve health or reduce obesity are easier for people who feel in control and in good psychosocial condition, lessening the burdens of low social status and relative poverty may make an important contribution both to better health and to a reduction of obesity' (p. 673).

The Marmot Review (2010) *Fair Society, Healthy Lives* was set up to consider health and wellbeing in England post-2010. It identified some pressing concerns, including the following.

- Reducing health inequalities is a matter of fairness and social justice. Many people – currently dying prematurely each year as a result of health inequalities – would otherwise have enjoyed between 1.3 and 2.5 million cumulative extra years of life.

- There is a social gradient influencing wellbeing, as the lower a person's social position, the more their health worsens. Action should focus on reducing this iniquitous gradient.
- Health inequalities result from social inequalities. This requires action across all the social determinants of health and wellbeing.
- Focusing solely on the most disadvantaged will not reduce health inequalities sufficiently. To reduce the steepness of the social gradient in health, actions must be universal but with a scale and intensity proportionate to the level of disadvantage, i.e. a concept of 'proportionate universalism'.
- Action taken to reduce health inequalities will benefit society. It will have economic benefits in reducing losses from illness associated with health inequalities, which account for productivity losses, reduced tax revenue, higher welfare payments and increased treatment costs.
- Economic growth is not the most important measure of success. Fair distribution of health, wellbeing and sustainability are important social goals; hence, tackling social inequalities in health and tackling climate change must go together.
- Reducing health inequalities requires action on six policy objectives:
  - giving every child the best start in life;
  - enabling all children, young people and adults to maximise their capabilities and have control over their lives;
  - creating fair employment and good work for all;
  - ensuring a healthy standard of living for all;
  - developing healthy and sustainable places and communities;
  - strengthening the role and impact of ill health prevention.
- Delivering these policy objectives requires action by central and local government, NHS, third and private sectors and community groups. National policies will not work without effective local delivery systems focused on health equity in all policies.
- Effective local delivery requires effective participatory decision making at local level. This can only happen by empowering individuals and local communities.

Given this context described by Marmot and the escalation of lifestyle-related conditions that mediate against wellbeing fulfilment, Evans (2004) identifies this as a tension for public health practice, between those having to embrace a neo-liberal 'free-market' approach – characterised by an individualised behavioural focus – and by practitioners advocating collective action that seeks to address wider aspects of community wellbeing.

The ideological context for public health promotion – and wellbeing approaches – is never static, yet much practice is premised on long-standing values and assumptions. The *Fair Society, Healthy Lives* findings are similar to certain core elements outlined by Tones and Tilford (1994) suggestive of highly traditional behavioural approaches to promoting and preserving wellbeing, which gained popularity from the 1970s. They identified similar facets for promoting wellbeing, comprising:

- enhancing overall quality of life;
- achieving positive health status, reached by addressing fundamental health inequalities;
- supporting more equitable distribution of resources to empower communities;
- employing principles of enablement and cooperation;
- recognising that wellbeing is determined by wider societal factors over which the individual has little control;
- developing mainstream healthy public policy strategies;
- going far beyond the confines of medicalisation.

Orme *et al.* (2007) note that public health practice operates in an increasingly fragmentary 'neo-liberal' world in which there is a multiplicity of wellbeing definitions, constructions and frameworks of analysis that arguably create schisms and uncertainty. Callinicos (2003) notes a global shift in political theorising that has affected UK approaches during the latter part of the twentieth century and beyond. He contends: 'It is indeed a peculiar kind of internationalism that leaves peoples free to choose the "single sustainable model of national success" – American-style laissez-faire capitalism' (p. 29). This led to the adoption and repackaging across Europe of hitherto right-wing concepts of freedom, liberty and individualism into everyday life at an unprecedented level. The UK economy now embraces key facets of a neo-liberal economy as part of an ongoing pragmatic approach to 'modernisation', especially concerning the reorienting of public services.

The significance of neo-liberalism to the wellbeing agenda

Present-day public health promoting practice has to operate within this fragmented context, which mediates society and, crucially, everyday wellbeing choices. According to Olssen and Peters (2005), central notions underpinning neo-liberalism include the following characteristics.

- Promoting the concept of global choice for individuals, organisations and multinational corporations. Committed to free trade solutions and not reliant upon subsidies or other forms of state-imposed protection or support.

- Privileging individualism, in which self-interest prevails. This views individuals as economically self-interested subjects; hence, the best judges of their own interests and needs.
- More regulation, audit and public accountability of professional roles. The consequence is to view all working relations as competitive hierarchies, which redefine accountability in terms of outputs, cost and quality.
- Minimising the role played by the state in everyday life and prioritising a commitment to free-market economics, rather than state bureaucracies.

The possible impact of neo-liberalism on wellbeing

Positioning neo-liberalism as one of the key global economic drivers has resulted in fragmentation and devolution of mainstream health services. This is characterised by moving away from positioning individuals as passive clients or patients, towards one in which seductive notions of 'active consumers' prevail. Hence, there is an ideological tension that public health initiatives need to acknowledge, both in terms of behavioural interventions to enhance wellbeing and in addressing health inequalities. In behavioural terms, individuals now live in a globalised neo-liberal climate in which self-interest (for those with the power to exert it) prevails; therefore, urging people to stay healthy – for the collective good of all – is becoming problematic and holds less significance for individuals, yet much public health is based on this premise. Furthermore, as the emerging neo-liberal citizens increasingly resent state interference, they are even less likely to comply with state-sponsored public health. Jones-Devitt and Smith (2007) suggest that such non-compliance will continue to escalate as the erosion between public, private and third-sector agencies for health services continues to blur.

Nafstad *et al.* (2007) note that this has led to an attrition of social welfare models of state intervention alongside the sanctioning of social inequalities. They argue that:

This ideology generally presumes that people's psyche amounts to little more than the single individual's freedom to choose and compete in order to maximise the possession of one's own material and non-material goods. People are primarily conceptualised as entirely self-interested, competitive and independent individuals, in the end driven by social greed ... this variant of modern capitalist ideology creates values that concentrate wealth and power in the hands of few, thereby legitimising social inequalities. (p. 316)

Bambra, Fox and Scott-Samuel (2003) argue that the lived reality of neo-liberalism, circa twenty-first century, represents: 'The imposition of a neo-liberal ideology and economics that systematically neglects the basic needs of the disadvantaged in its pursuit of the accumulation of money, property and natural resources. This is resulting in a widening gap in wealth, health and quality of life' (p. 23).

Activity 2.2 Considering the possible impact of neo-liberalism on wellbeing

Consider the four key elements of neo-liberalism, identified above by Olssen and Peters (2005). How much influence do these have on everyday life? How can effective wellbeing approaches be developed that acknowledge an increasing culture of individualism, while still enhancing overall social cohesion?

DEVELOPING EFFECTIVE WELLBEING PROMOTION PRACTICE

Given the changing context for wellbeing, Checkland (2004) notes that practitioners need to act as autonomous, multiskilled inter-sectoral workers, while operating within increasingly regulated frameworks. They also need to manage the changed expectations of the individual 'citizen', in which the diversification and fragmentation of public health has gained further momentum, with wellbeing becoming ever-expansive and intertwined within many facets of ordinary life.

Within a culture of growing individualism, challenges to medical ownership of health have accelerated due to reduction of acute disease incidence and wider public access to web-based information, alongside the ascendancy of chronic and enduring illnesses that make long-term conditions – and resultant sub-maximal expectations of wellbeing – part of many people's everyday lives. Given these constraints, it is optimistic to expect public health to effectively address both the UK inequalities chasm while developing salutogenic approaches for overall wellbeing.

A pragmatic approach is offered within the New Economics Foundation/ Nottingham City Council Case Study below that could prove cost-effective and more engaging when targeted at specific elements of the population. It feeds into the zeitgeist of neo-liberalism by providing measurable outcomes of wellbeing. (See also the NICE guidelines for targeted wellbeing interventions as part of Mental Wellbeing and Older People resources at: **http://guidance.nice.org.uk/PH16/**) The approach shown in the case study below could make public health tangible within the individual's everyday existence, while enhancing overall wellbeing.

Case Study 2.1 New Economics Foundation and Nottingham City Council

The following study highlights why a salutogenic approach – as advocated by Antonovsky – can be more effective than those focusing on health and wellbeing 'deficits'. It resulted in the development of a two-dimensional model of wellbeing, which focused on life satisfaction and personal development. More importantly, the multidimensional wellbeing model and overall approach could be scaled up according to need and across all age ranges and genders.

As defined by the Local Government Act (2000) and latterly by Dolan *et al.* (2006), local councils have gained new powers to promote economic, social and environmentally sustainable wellbeing. Operationalising local wellbeing policy has led to questions about how to define, promote and measure wellbeing effectively. Hence, the New Economics Foundation and Nottingham City Council undertook a pilot project to measure the wellbeing of young people in Nottingham. The aims of the collaborative project were to:

- explore ways of using local authority powers to promote wellbeing;
- examine and test out theories of wellbeing;
- learn more about ways to measure wellbeing, particularly using multidimensional approaches;
- illuminate factors influencing young people's wellbeing;
- understand how such research can assist policy making.

The project used a multidimensional model of wellbeing for the theoretical base, while also looking at new ways of using the local government wellbeing powers. Over 1000 children and young people in Nottingham, aged 7–19, were surveyed. Questionnaires were designed to enable scales of life satisfaction and curiosity –

used as an indicator of children's capacity for personal development – to be measured and calculated. Other scales used included those which assessed:

- children's satisfaction with different aspects of their lives, such as their families, friendships, neighbourhoods and schools;
- children's tendency to display characteristics of 'pro-social' behaviour and favourite weekly activities.

One of the key findings of the study identified that there is more to life than satisfaction alone. Many interventions measure wellbeing only in terms of people's satisfaction, commonly called 'life satisfaction'. The research from this study confirms the view that there is at least another dimension to wellbeing, concerning 'personal development', which has important implications for future wellbeing research and policy making. This second dimension of wellbeing is related particularly to long-term health outcomes and to the ability to cope flexibly and creatively with life's challenges, exemplified in the two-dimensional model below.

Core elements of a two-dimensional model of wellbeing

1. Life satisfaction – capturing satisfaction, pleasure, enjoyment and contentment.
2. Personal development – capturing curiosity, enthusiasm, absorption, flow, exploration, commitment, creative challenge and meaningfulness.

Measuring the wellbeing of young people created a new picture of Nottingham, which complemented but also contrasted with that already known. Historically, local authorities tend to focus on problems and deficits – such as anti-social behaviour, crime or ill-health – rather than focusing on finding out what helps to make people's lives meaningful. The latter approach could be more effective in tackling some of the problems directly. This small study indicates that focusing attention on young people's wellbeing – from a salutogenic perspective – illustrates some key policy areas and activities that promote sustainable wellbeing.

The study also shows that the process of using shared indicators for evidence across local government can begin to transform ways in which local government operates. It also highlights key questions that all wellbeing approaches should explore. Therefore, wellbeing indicators serve as a practical way in which the 'power of wellbeing' can be used to join local services and functions to better meet people's needs within communities.

Source: New Economic Foundation (2004) *The Potential and Power of Wellbeing Indicators: measuring young people's wellbeing in Nottingham*. London: NEF

Universalism

The Marmot Review (2010) notion of 'proportionate universalism' as a means to enhancing wellbeing is not new. Thomas More (1516) presented a more radical notion of universalism in which he explored the conceptualisation of a 'utopian' society without private property as idyllic. Wilkinson (2005) concurs that more equal societies equate to far healthier ones. In the twenty-first century, some interesting notions of wellbeing linked to income distribution abound. Shah and Marks (2004) advocate a universal approach via the concept of a 'Citizen's Income', which they define as:

A tax-free income paid to all people (including children) by the State regardless of employment status or social circumstance. It would enable people to make wider choices about how to allocate their time between employment, unpaid work, parenting and leisure ... basic income would have important redistributive effects. It would also promote employment as it would reduce the level at which paid work becomes worthwhile: the present benefits system discourages work as moving from unemployment to paid work may bring very little rise in disposable income after travel costs, childcare, etc., are taken into account (p.10).

While Shah and Marks contend that wellbeing would be enhanced by much flatter socio-economic structures, attempting to engineer such radical social equality is far more difficult in a neo-liberal context, underpinned by growing self-interest, laissez-faire attitudes to social relations and the erosion of the welfare state.

Activity 2.3 PEST analysis for wellbeing

Complete a PEST analysis for wellbeing, drawing on the chapter discourse. PEST provides a framework for assessment of Political, Economic, Socio-cultural and Technological factors that can influence wellbeing approaches. Refer to Table 2.1 to assist your thinking.

Political The prevailing policy drivers and ideological approaches for wellbeing.	**Economic** The subtext for much decision making and prioritisation of wellbeing initiatives.
Socio-cultural Society's norms and cultural expectations of wellbeing.	**Technological** Influence of new technological advances for wellbeing enhancement.

Table 2.1 PEST framework for wellbeing

Feasible wellbeing approaches?

In earlier versions of public health promotion, described above by Tones and Tilford (1994), the process was paramount, rather than the results. Contemporary wellbeing models can provide measurable indicators and outcomes as described in the case study above. These also resonate with the plethora of tools and cost-effective approaches available from the National Institute for Health and Clinical Excellence (NICE). This approach aligns with the recent development of 'Nudge Theory' in which behavioural economics is combined with psychological theories of motivation. Thaler and Sunstein (2009) contend that people do not always make the best decisions independently when faced with many choices. They argue that people often require assistance rather than coercion. They describe the difference between the two concepts by introducing the notion of 'libertarian paternalism', indicating that those choices deemed more positive should be highlighted and encouraged:

> Libertarian paternalists want to make it easy for people to go their own way; they do not want to burden those who want to exercise their freedom. The paternalistic aspect lies in the claim that it is legitimate for choice architects to try to influence people's behavior

in order to make their lives longer, healthier and better ... we argue for self-conscious efforts, by institutions in the private sector and also by government, to steer people's choices in directions that will improve their lives (p. 5).

One further 'unthinkable' notion – drawing heavily upon Nudge Theory – involves using direct-payments models as a way of offering a more transparent approach to achieving wellbeing via targeted behavioural interventions and income redistribution. This would be embedded within acceptable neo-liberal parameters of 'personalisation' which have become the progressive model for social care. A direct-payments model of wellbeing may have further appeal as it:

- **Reduces the overt control of professionals**: relating to the spending choices of targeted individuals. In more conventional wellbeing approaches, access to capital and resources are determined only by professionals.
- **Redirects finite public health resources**: moving away from the middle-class 'worried well' to those who really need it. Any middle-class backlash would be offset by reducing the level of basic income tax for those who stay well. This could be made due to savings from enhancing the wellbeing of the poor, as reduced illnesses and lower hospitalisation rates could provide longer-term financial benefits for the economy as defined by the Marmot Review (2010) via the concept of proportionate universalism.
- **Makes public health mainstream**: regular direct payments will make a tangible difference to the lives of the poorest in ways that other forms of public health intervention cannot achieve, lifting participants out of poverty and into wellbeing.

CONCLUSION

This chapter has presented some of the complexities when trying to disaggregate wellbeing from the concept of health. Regardless of political hue, it is clear that wellbeing interventions will have to demonstrate measurable and evidence-based outcomes if they are to be deemed effective in an increasingly audited and outputs-driven climate for health and social care. The influence of neo-liberalism has to be acknowledged in practical terms by public health practitioners, even if this results in an inevitable reduction of large-scale social justice models for wellbeing. This chapter argues that many facets of neo-liberalism add to the burden of overall inequality for the poorest in UK society, yet there is little option but to embrace some aspects of this prevailing zeitgeist by positioning forms of pragmatic public health (see the NEF case study, Nudge Theory and direct payments referred to above) that capture the ethos, while still prioritising the neediest members of society. Otherwise, public health approaches for wellbeing will be further marginalised as ineffective and obsolete phenomena.

Further reading

Foley, M. (2010) *The Age of Absurdity*. London: Simon and Schuster UK Ltd

A very provocative text offering interesting insights into why overall fulfilment becomes more elusive in contemporary society.

Websites

New Economics Foundation: **www.neweconomics.org/programmes/ wellbeing**

A non-party politically aligned think tank incorporating the Centre for Wellbeing, which showcases research, policies, measurement tools and actions aimed at increasing wellbeing.

Chapter 3

Ethics and Wellbeing

Nevin Mehmet

Learning outcomes

In this chapter you will learn how to:

- relate ethical theories and concepts to wellbeing;

- analyse the differences between health and wellbeing using ethical concepts;

- discuss what happiness means in an ethical context;

- analyse the role of personal responsibility in respect of wellbeing.

This chapter will focus on the ways in which ethical theories and philosophical concepts are related to wellbeing. It provides an overview of how ancient philosophy teachings from the likes of Socrates, Plato and Aristotle have shaped the way in which the concept of human wellbeing is viewed and what it means to live 'the good life'. This chapter will explore the concept of happiness and explore some of the main ethical theories and concepts of wellbeing.

INTRODUCTION

Ethics, or the more commonly used term 'normative ethics', addresses questions about morality in that it attempts to define what is good and evil, right and wrong, justice and virtue. Ethics is a part of philosophical thinking. Philosophy dates back to ancient civilisation and has provided a platform for moral reasoning and philosophical understanding of how one should live.

Modern philosophers or ethicists have contributed two main ethical theories to the development of health care thinking, namely utilitarianism and deontology. Utilitarianism is a doctrine proposed by Jeremy Bentham (1748–1832) and later by John Stuart Mill (1806–76), whereby an action is morally good if it produces the greatest amount of good or pleasure for the greatest number of people. Deontology (*deon* meaning 'duty') proposes that it is the moral intention of the agent that makes the action right or wrong. According to Immanuel Kant (1734–1804), we have a moral duty within society to act in a morally right way. Kant established a set of universal laws whereby a moral action was either right or wrong in a more universal context (applicable to all). Using this approach, Beauchamp and Childress (2001) established a set of principles (autonomy, beneficence, non-maleficence and justice) that originate in deontology theory. These two main ethical theories and principles provide a framework for critical thinking, and provide a structure for the analysis of difficult moral dilemmas and situations that can arise within a health care setting.

Virtue ethics arose from the work of the ancient philosopher Socrates and was then developed by Plato and, more extensively, through the work of Aristotle. This theory focuses the attention on character rather than actions (though that's not to say actions are not considered), and particularly focuses on the virtues of the individual. This will be discussed further within this chapter. However, Socrates, Plato and Aristotle, using the underpinnings of Virtue Theory, sought to answer the complexities of wellbeing, and what it means to live a 'good life'.

Within the ethical context, wellbeing, according to Crisp (2008), is most commonly used within philosophy to describe what is good for a person, and this question is of great importance within moral philosophy. Buchanan (2000) poignantly defines wellbeing in terms of integrity, of living one's life in accordance with values that matter. It is the constant striving to see more clearly the values that define us as human beings, the kind of person one wants to be and the kind of society one wants to live in that enables us to live a 'well' life. Although different values may well conflict with one another, and different individuals may express differing values that give their lives meaning, purpose and happiness, nevertheless it is a life based on integrity (common value) that, according to Buchanan (2000), enhances our wellbeing.

Note that the definition of wellbeing discussed within this chapter is in the context of philosophical questions and does not replace those outlined in other chapters in this book.

THE DIFFERENCES BETWEEN HEALTH AND WELLBEING

The terms and meanings of 'health' and 'wellbeing' have become conflated in modern use, despite their being conceptually distinct. Health is now an integral part of popular concerns, with copious reading material and the advertising of books on diet, exercise, stress, recovery, vitamins and biofeedback. Health books have replaced books on the philosophy of the good life and we have reduced the concept and idea of the human good life to physical fitness and to the regimented rituals of diet and exercise. The WHO definition of 'health' is rather static and provides an impoverished notion of what constitutes wellbeing. Crisp (2008) states that the philosophical term 'wellbeing' is far broader, encapsulating concepts that relate more individualistically to how well a person's life is lived. Crisp views health as constituent of wellbeing and, more importantly, that health is not all that enhances wellbeing. To confirm the challenges now facing the field of philosophy, we need to rethink the terms and conditions of wellbeing that go beyond the regimes of physical fitness and beauty rituals.

Aristotle made a consistent distinction between 'health' and 'wellbeing'. Health (*halos*) referred to the biological functioning, but 'wellbeing' was denoted by the Greek term *eudemonia*, which may also be translated as 'flourishing', 'happiness', 'blessedness' or 'prosperity'. In Aristotle's writings, wellbeing is the ultimate good, the *telos* ('end' or 'goal') of all human activity, which is guided by our ability to reason, and it is therefore categorically distinct from all 'natural goods' such as health and wealth. According to Aristotle, health is too dependent on fate, fortune or luck; it was unthinkable to Aristotle to leave the prospects of living a good life to chance. Health and wealth were mere instrumental goods. Placing a higher priority on pursuing wealth or health than on living an honourable life could be harmful, both materially and morally. Wellbeing is what he saw as the highest goal of human activity; this should be the pursuit towards which all intentional, purposive and reasoned actions are directed.

Therefore, according to Aristotle, the *telos* of rational human activity is to bring about wellbeing, happiness and the 'good life' for human beings, but what is the 'good life'? Aristotle characterised human flourishing as a life of excelling in values that are distinctively human. In his words, 'How should a human being live? In accordance with all the forms of good functioning that makes up a good human life' (Aristotle, 1985).

Activity 3.1 Reflection

- What do you think Aristotle meant in the quote above?
- Aristotle used the analogy of a knife to describe human functioning. We call a knife a good knife if it cuts well, because this is the function of the knife. So we could, by comparison, call a human life a good life if it did that which is a defining function. What do you think this means?
- Write a list of what you think makes us human and what are our 'functions'.

This distinction between health and wellbeing offers an alternative to the health status model of wellbeing that has dominated health promotion, and this enables us to understand how health professionals may have confused a state of physical fitness with the ideal of wellbeing. In a health context, this distinction enables us to understand individuals who may suffer a disease but who we would still regard as living well. For example, a woman who is diagnosed with breast cancer who peacefully approaches her own death with the support of the family might be said to be 'well', despite the fact that she is facing death.

Using this example, it is fair to question whether we see health as a descriptive term or a normative concept. Are we well when we measure up to a set of clearly defined indicators, or does the concept refer to an evolving understanding of the values and ideals now packed into the term 'wellbeing'? Is there a connection between how health and wellbeing are viewed by society and by individuals? As a society in the UK we have a fairly passionate regard for physical fitness and this is evident in the cornucopia of workout videos, gym memberships, sports clothing and smoking bans while, at the same time, we have among the highest rates of violence, drug abuse, STDs and obesity in the world. What does all this suggest to us about society's concept of wellbeing?

It is clear that defining distinctive concepts of health and wellbeing that evaluate the conceptual view of promoting individual health, not by a set of risk factors, but through a shift in our approach, would entail us viewing wellbeing as a process of living well through the engagement in social practices that embody a set of common values.

THEORIES OF WELLBEING

Before the concept of happiness can be discussed, we should explore the theories of wellbeing that provide the basis of the philosophical underpinning from which happiness is derived when discussing living a 'happy' or a 'good' life. Parfit (1984) divides theories of wellbeing into three types:

- hedonistic;
- desire;
- list theories.

Hedonistic wellbeing

Hedonism identifies wellbeing with pleasure; it is primarily concerned with balancing the greatest pleasures. Socrates was the first philosopher to discuss hedonism in relation to obtaining happiness. This view was extended by Bentham (1969), cited in Haybron (2008), who said that nature placed human beings under the governance of two supreme masters, pain and pleasure, and, by balancing these two experiences, a hedonist will seek experiences that value pleasure over pain. The more pleasantness one can pack into one's life the better it will be, and the more painfulness one encounters the worse it will be, and the duration and intensity of these experiences will enable the individual to measure their value.

Activity 3.2 Nozick's objection

Imagine a machine that you could be plugged into for the rest of your life. This machine would give you experiences of whatever kind you thought most valuable or enjoyable (writing a novel, playing sports, attending concerts, etc.). You would not know you were plugged into the machine and there is no worry about machine failure. Once plugged in you would remain there for the rest of your life.

1. What would you plug into?
2. How would this benefit your wellbeing?
3. Is this a man-made experience? A Virtual World?
4. Would this affect the value of your experiences?

According to Crisp (2003) and Haybron (2008), the attraction of this view is that it accommodates the plausible thought that if anything matters for individual welfare it is the pleasantness of life experiences. Despite the attractiveness of this theory, a serious objection by Nozick (1974), based on the 'experience machine' analogy (see Activity 3.2), still forms the basis of rejection of this theory by modern-day philosophers.

Desire

Desire theories identify wellbeing with the satisfaction of individual desires. A common version of desire theory is 'informed desire', whereby an individual is informed about all the facts of a particular desire, thus providing a platform for rationality and reflection. The positive aspect of this theory is the flexibility of acknowledging the varying desires that individuals seek, particularly in a changing society where desires change with modernity. The problem with this approach is the reliance on a specific form of individual pleasure in order to achieve wellbeing that could have the potential to harm other individuals even if informed desire is exercised. Aristotle, cited in Crisp (2008), states that relying on a theory whereby we seek to uphold our desires is somewhat problematic, irrespective of whether those desires are informed or not.

Objective list theories

Objective list theories are understood as theories that create lists of what constitutes wellbeing, which consist neither merely in pleasurable experience nor in desire satisfaction. These lists would include friendship, knowledge, accomplishments, etc. Therefore what should go on the list? Haybron (2008) and Crisp (2003) point out that every good should be part of the list, and what is to be part of an individual's list is based on intuition and reflective judgement. Using a more rationalist approach, this encompasses other external pleasures such as friendship and relationships.

An objection to list theories is that they are limited, as they claim that certain things are good for individuals even if they may not enjoy them: for example, including friendship when one might find it more pleasurable to live life alone. The point is that the list theories have a tendency to assume the common 'good' that individuals should adopt, though, on the other hand, list theories may allow for exploration of the values or 'goods' that we all deem to be universally valid.

Although there are objections to these theories of wellbeing, what is evident is that, by taking a more generalist approach, one can assume that modern-day society is adopting a hedonistic and desire satisfaction approach to happiness. There are obviously negative consequences of this constant seeking of pleasures: for example, the increase in STDs, alcoholism, drug abuse and violent behaviour. Nevertheless, the objective list theory does encompass values and by using this theory a more universal approach to happiness can be further explored.

VIRTUE ETHICS

> ... we must look more closely at the matter, since what is at stake is far from insignificant: it is how one should live one's life. (Plato, 1992, cited in Haybron, 2008, p. 6)

Virtue Ethics (VE) are concerned with an individual's character, whereas with consequentialism and deontology it is the individual's actions that are of importance (Macintyre, 2007). For Virtue theorists the central question of morality is 'What kind of person ought I to be?' and not 'What ought I to do?' Arguably, due to its agent-based nature, virtue can be seen as the heart of our moral reasoning as it is the character of the person that can determine which action to take, irrespective of duty/ obligation or aspiring to the greater good. As human beings we have the ability to reason, tempered by our emotional reactions, that enables us to make judgements about our actions. Moreover, it is the habitual practice of our experiences and behaviours that can determine how we develop good characteristics and that enables us to act in a morally good way (Gardiner, 2003). The character of the moral agent is pivotal in VE and this is what sets VE apart from deontology and consequentialism.

Historically VE began with the Greek philosophers Socrates, Plato and Aristotle. Their search for the elements that made a person good was not based on the way a person acted but on what sort of characteristics a person had. For example, an honest person is not just someone who performs honest acts, it is a disposition that is ingrained in the individual (Macintyre, 2007). Additionally, Aristotle, the father of VE, outlined four cardinal virtues:

- courage/fortitude;
- temperance;
- prudence/wisdom;
- justice.

Aristotle considered these virtues to be of the utmost importance in an individual's morality (Slote, 2001). Over time the habitual practice of these virtues enables an individual to act in a good way when confronted with a moral dilemma. Aristotle termed this phrenesis or 'practical wisdom'. An ability to be virtuous, by the exercising of the virtues together rather than in isolation, leads to eudemonia or 'human flourishing' or 'wellbeing'. The question that then arises is how do we act virtuously and, most importantly, how do you know when you have acted virtuously? The 'doctrine of the mean' is that someone's character lies between two states of the given virtue. For example, if we look at courage as being a virtue then vices would be either a deficiency of virtue, i.e. acting in a cowardly way, or an excess of the virtue, i.e. being foolhardy. Therefore, to be courageous would be the mean between these two states. For example, defending your home against an intruder is courageous, but if you are outnumbered or your life is in danger then, arguably, Aristotle would interpret this as being foolhardy and not courageous.

As society norms have evolved and changed over time, what we deem as virtuous has also evolved. Although some universal virtues have stayed the same, for example, honesty, justice and courage, some of the other virtues have been driven out by our society norms. Chastity, for example, is no longer considered a virtue. Modern-day ethicists such as Rachels (1999) and Hursthouse (1999) identify benevolence, civility, self-control, compassion and kindness as an evolution of the original virtues. However, they are still based on interpretations of the cardinal virtues, so many different formulations do exist, but the fundamental virtues still remain.

Activity 3.3 Reflection

- What do you think about Aristotle's virtues?
- How are these virtues learned, imparted or acquired?
- Do you think that some of these virtues have been lost in today's society and, if so, which ones? Should they be acquired again?

HAPPINESS VS EUDEMONIA

> They have their little pleasures for the day and their little pleasure for the night: but they respect health. 'We have discovered happiness' say the Ultimate men and blink. (Friedrich Nietzsche, cited in Buchanan, 2000, p. 102)

Nietzsche's quote distinguishes 'Ultimate men' as individuals who think they have discovered happiness through little pleasures but who still maintain the concept that having health is a state of wellbeing. Nietzsche and Aristotle disagree about this, as a heavy preoccupation with physical fitness can become as harmful to wellbeing, both materially and morally, as if we neglected physical fitness altogether. This follows on from the concept discussed above regarding the distinction between health and wellbeing, i.e. that to be in a state of wellness and to feel happiness goes beyond physical fitness, materialism and wealth.

What needs to be established here is what we mean by happiness and we need to keep in mind the different ways in which happiness is defined by different authors. A generally accepted basic view is that happiness is often referred to as a short-lived state of an individual, through a feeling of contentment (Haybron, 2008). This approach forms the basis of philosophical understandings of wellbeing, particularly when comparisons are drawn between living an eudemonian life as opposed to a happy life.

Subjective wellbeing

Deci and Ryan (2008) discuss the concept that wellbeing can be thought of as falling into two distinct traditions, the hedonistic state where the focus is on happiness, and eudemonia, focusing on living well in a more full and satisfying way, although this is based on subjectivism. Vigorous study by Diener (1984) led to the exploration of subjective wellbeing as a term that is often referred to within contemporary research into wellbeing. In Diener's view, wellbeing is considered to be subjective (SWB) because individuals evaluate for themselves, in a more general way, the degree to which they experience a sense of wellness. Experiencing high levels of positive experiences rather than negative experiences, and having a high level of satisfaction within one's life, leads to 'happiness'.

Subjective wellbeing (SWB) as referred to by Kahneman *et al.* (1999) has been closely associated with the hedonistic view of wellbeing, as its central focus is evaluating positive experiences of pleasure. However, what is interesting to note is that many philosophers and researchers in the field of wellbeing draw upon a more Aristotelian view of wellbeing and eudemonia, in that happiness alone does not constitute wellbeing. Yes, one does need to experience feelings of happiness. But though individuals may report feeling happy or being positively satisfied, this does not necessarily mean that they are psychologically well.

Waterman (1993) stated that wellbeing should not be thought of as an outcome or an end state, but rather a process of fulfilling one's virtuous potentials and living as one was inherently intended to live (we can see this example through Aristotle's analogy of a good knife). Seeking happiness as an outcome to wellbeing through hedonistic pleasure has its problems, as it becomes a state of seeking pleasures or gratifications that may have undesired consequences not only for the specific individual but society as a whole. For example, living a promiscuous life and constantly seeking the feeling of this pleasure may result in the contraction of STDs if precautions are not taken. One could also draw on the examples of not living a virtuous life and not exercising temperance.

Wellbeing and desire satisfaction

The same evaluation may be applied to desire satisfaction as a way of trying to obtain happiness as a state of wellbeing. If we strive to obtain our set desires this again may have detrimental effects collectively and individually as, without exercising judgement and applying a rationale to what constitutes 'useful' desires, desire satisfaction may actually result in unhappiness.

The objective list theories encompass other aspects that one would expect to describe in terms of values such as friendship, relationships, socialisation and accomplishments, and a sense of achievement. Although certain aspects of individuals' lists may be somewhat different, this theory does provide a much stronger understanding of accepting our social needs when seeking 'happiness'. Aristotle's vision of the 'good life' states that humans have the power to evaluate desires and to regard some as desirable and some as undesirable, and this is what makes human beings distinctive. It is the ability to evaluate and exercise judgements that can truly lead individuals to understand what 'happiness' is (Slote, 2001).

Although in some literature eudemonia is used as a synonym for happiness and wellbeing, this can be somewhat problematic. Eudemonia is more concerned with leading a eudemonian life by exercising virtues that in time become habitual through *phrenesis* or 'practical wisdom'.

Happiness, as we have seen, is subjective irrespective of the theories that are used to determine the term 'happiness'. It is a subjective feeling and therefore turns the focus onto specific internal needs. Interestingly, Aristotle had no theory of happiness, only a theory of wellbeing. For Aristotle, to define the concept of happiness would only go against living an eudemonian life, in that the focus would be on simply obtaining pleasures but not necessarily living a good life. Happiness was a state of being and not a state of living so, according to Aristotle, it is only by leading an eudemonian life that humans can flourish and live a life of wellbeing.

PERSONAL RESPONSIBILITY

A concept that is closely related to eudemonia is autonomy. Ryan and Deci (2001) define autonomy within this context as having the experience of choice to endorse one's actions at the highest level of reflection. Aristotle emphasised choice and suggested that virtue, which is central to eudemonia, involves making the right choices; an individual chooses to act virtuously.

As a society are we living a hedonistic life? Are we seeking pleasures that make us happy? Is this wellbeing? We have recently (2010) experienced a period of recession and, although there are strong economic debates about why this has occurred, the question in philosophical terms is, are we living beyond our means? By trying to be happy have we been driven to seek happiness in materialism and possessions? Have we been using what can be considered hedonistic pleasures to try to obtain a 'good life'? A strong objection to pursuing hedonism for happiness or a 'good life' is that, instead of enjoying pleasurable experiences and accepting that this is all they are – just a pleasurable experience – it becomes a habit of collecting pleasures to try to maximise happiness. There is therefore a loss of understanding of the intrinsic value of some activities because, by maximising our own pleasures, we become unable to immerse ourselves in activities such as reading and playing sports that are in themselves valuable, but that also provide pleasure. It is only through taking personal responsibility for the evaluation of these activities that we achieve the understanding that these activities are independently valuable, irrespective of the pleasure we gain from them, and only once we understand this can we begin to understand the meaning of wellbeing.

Nussbaum (1994) held the view that the upbringing of our children and adolescents is deformed in various ways by false views about what matters in life – excessive emphasis is placed on money, competition and status, and placing value on materialism, rather than placing value on personal attributes and how to lead a 'good life'. Plato stated that it is impossible to heal the body without at the same time treating the soul. Modern scientific medicine has conquered most infectious diseases and many types of biological breakdowns, but it is still ill-equipped for the task of diagnosing and treating ailments of the soul; modern medicine does not have an answer for the problems that stem from our desires and the choices we make about how we want to live our lives (Buchanan, 2000). We have to take personal responsibility for the health of our souls.

Case study and activity 3.4 Applying philosophical approaches to real-life scenarios

Suzan is a 25 year-old who works in a fulltime administrative position. Suzan lives with her parents and a year ago she split up with her boyfriend of two years. Since then she has been on a downward spiral of late nights, alcohol and drug abuse and has had over 50 sexual partners. One night Suzan is taken to A&E following a night of heavy drinking – one of her many admissions to A&E. The A&E staff have recommended that she sees a counsellor so, following a consultation with her GP, she has been referred to the practice counsellor and Suzan has agreed to this.

- What aspects indicate that Suzan is happy or unhappy?
- What aspects of Suzan's life may be attributed to eudemonia?
- What options are available to Suzan?
- What virtues and values are missing from Suzan's life?

Exercising mindfulness and personal responsibility uses Aristotle's approach in that he states that we should look after ourselves before we think about others. If we all exercise virtues then we benefit, and our community and society also benefit in the development of wellbeing. Virtues are not unattainable goals but well within our reach. Although, to some extent, we are conditioned by the society we live in, at some point we have to assume responsibility for the habits we acquire. See Chapter 7 on spirituality, which discusses the importance of personal responsibility and wellbeing.

CONCLUSION

This chapter has explored the ethical theories and concepts that address what we mean by wellbeing. For example, the belief that being healthy constitutes wellbeing is a misconception. What has been discussed in this chapter is the constant struggle that philosophers and ethicists face when discussing the notion of happiness in relation to wellbeing. Although, to some extent, wellbeing is subjective, particularly when the focus is on happiness, it is through an analysis of what constitutes a 'good life' that we can begin to explore the concept of wellbeing. Aristotle retained his view that it is only by exercising virtues that we can begin to lead a eudemonian life that results in true wellbeing. It is only through personal responsibility and through analysis of ourselves that we can begin to determine our own wellbeing. Temperance or, to use a more modern term, 'mindfulness' encourages individuals not to take a hedonistic approach to happiness but, rather, it is through analysis and contemplation of values and, more importantly, society's values, that we can achieve true wellbeing. Indeed, it is only by focusing on our inner selves and our own wellbeing that we can truly flourish within society.

Further reading

Bond E.J. (1996) *Ethics and Human Well Being: An Introduction to Moral Philosophy*. London: Blackwell Publishers

An ideal introduction to moral philosophy as it deals with the philosophical theories that often lie behind everyday opinions.

Chapter 4

Monitoring and Evaluating Wellbeing Projects

Carlos Moreno-Leguizamon and Clarence Spigner

Learning outcomes

In this chapter you will learn how to:

- distinguish two main approaches to monitoring and evaluation in terms of research and management functions;

- develop a workable characterisation of wellbeing when either monitoring or evaluating a project initiative;

- know why, what and how to monitor and evaluate a wellbeing project or initiative.

INTRODUCTION

The aim of this chapter is to present a framework for monitoring and evaluating wellbeing projects or initiatives. The chapter is organised in three parts. The first part presents and discusses two main monitoring and evaluation approaches, including their differences and pros and cons. The two approaches, a results-based management framework and outcome mapping, are currently being used by governments, multilateral and bilateral organisations, and research institutions to strengthen their capacity in terms of monitoring and evaluation. Due to growing pressure, as evidenced by the Millennium Development Goals (UN, 2010), there is an increasing emphasis on results, accountability and resources for both research and development projects and initiatives. Stakeholders in both developed and developing countries alike want to know how effectively projects or initiatives are contributing to making people's lives better. The wellbeing area is no exception. The second part of the chapter attempts to discuss and characterise the category of wellbeing as discussed by various discourses and researchers (Bakshi, 2007; Bourne, 2010; Cameron *et al.*, 2006; Diener, 2009; Dierich, 2007; NEF, 2004; Stecker, 2004; Wilkinson, 2007).

Material, mental, emotional, spiritual, psychological, economic and social wellbeing are, among others, the notions that one can come across when reviewing the literature on wellbeing. Characterising or categorising what is meant by the term wellbeing is important in order to know why, what and how to evaluate a project or an initiative (Bourne, 2010). The third part of the chapter focuses specifically on responding to the 'why, what and how' to monitor and evaluate projects. It is expected that professionals and students interested in wellbeing will be able to appreciate what monitoring and evaluation entails as managerial and research functions.

MONITORING AND EVALUATION AS RESEARCH AND MANAGEMENT FUNCTIONS

Currently, both monitoring and evaluation are considered not only research functions but also managerial functions that complement each other (UNDP, 2002). Thus, an effective project or initiative should ideally have a dialogue and interface between these two. First, the monitoring of a project or initiative should be carried out on a regular basis by its stakeholders as an internal self-assessment and reflection on how the project or initiative is performing. Second, the evaluation of a project or initiative should be carried out by an external reviewer or agent in relation to how the project or initiative is performing (mid-term evaluation) or has performed on its completion (final evaluation) or over the long term (impact evaluation).

Monitoring, defined generally, is understood both as an internal research and management function, undertaken to provide continuous indication – almost 'daily' – of the progress, or lack of it, of a project or initiative in terms of the achievement of aims (results) by its managers and stakeholders. Aims and results relate to the same concept of actions according to the results-based management approach. The only aspect that changes about them is that aims are written as future actions while results are actions that have been completed. Evaluation, on the other hand, is a time-bound process of researching the achievement of results of a project or initiative in a systematic way at its mid- and end-points, in order to assess the relevance and success of resulting changes (see Figure 4.1). Internationally there is almost a consensus among organisations such as the United Nations, the World Bank and the European Commission that the criteria for monitoring and evaluating a project or initiative should focus minimally on:

- **Relevance:** under this criterion we should assess issues such as whether the groups being targeted by the project or initiative are benefiting (monitoring) or have benefited (evaluation) directly or not, and whether the theme of the project or initiative maintains its relevance while the project or initiative is implemented (monitoring) or has been implemented (evaluation).
- **Performance**: under this criterion we should assess issues such as effectiveness or the extent to which the objectives or goal(s) of the project or initiative are being met (monitoring) or have been met (evaluation). Meanwhile, timeliness should be assessed by asking whether the project or initiative is doing the required things (monitoring) or has done the required things (evaluation) at the right moments in time. Lack of focus and delayed funding, for example, are among the most common indicators of poor performance in many projects and initiatives.

- **Success**: under this criterion we should assess issues such as impact (intended or unintended change of a problem or a reality), sustainability (financial or otherwise) and contribution to capacity building, so that the project or initiative stakeholders can continue alone, scaling out or up the work once the financial support has ended.

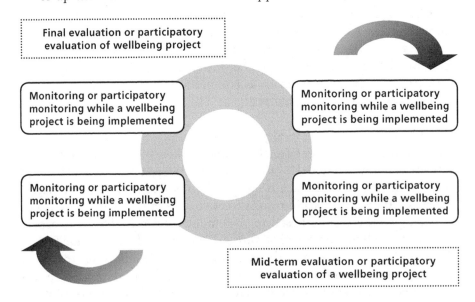

Figure 4.1 Illustrates monitoring and evaluation as research and managerial functions as they should occur in the cycle of a wellbeing project or initiative

Nowadays, in some open, innovative and democratically oriented institutions and organisations, managers prefer talking in terms of participatory monitoring and evaluation (Suarez-Herrera *et al.*, 2009). The first one is the same as monitoring but its meaning changes and becomes participatory when as many stakeholders as possible become engaged in the managerial and research process, especially the end-users or service users. In small- and mid-scale projects it is very good practice to assess whether what the project or initiative is doing makes sense to either only managers, funders or to all. In the case of evaluation and participatory evaluation the differences relate basically to who does the evaluation. If the end-users or customers are included, and their role of being the 'objects' of evaluation is modified to that of 'subjects' doing the evaluating, an evaluation is considered participatory. Furthermore, participatory and non-participatory evaluations currently include reflections by all stakeholders, but primarily policy makers, on the lessons learnt, since this should help them to avoid repeating the same mistakes and, therefore, save resources. The lack of reflection and failure to identify the lessons learnt are also, for example, common indicators of poor performance of many projects and initiatives.

Behind monitoring and evaluation, as both research and management functions, there is an assumed logic which it is important to address in order to understand what is expected when someone is confronted with the activity of either monitoring or evaluation. This model, as McCawley (1997) points out, basically represents a set of logical linkages between projects' or initiatives' resources (inputs), activities, results (outputs, outcomes and impacts), stakeholders and, finally, the short-, mid- and long-term impact in relation to a situation or problem (i.e. the project's or initiative's theme such as, for example, family wellbeing). Once it is understood that a project or initiative is underpinned by this logic, the identification of the basic critical measures of performance need to be set up (for example, relevance, performance and success, as discussed above) (McCawley, 1997).

The assumptions of the logical models could be criticised for their lack of flexibility and their tendency to miss important aspects of processes and relationships (Woodhill, 2005). An additional criticism is associated with the mechanistic assumption of the logical model – its implicit cause/effect model. The fact that X organisation or institution has supported a process of change in a community through a project or initiative does not necessarily mean that the change has occurred only because of that support. The impact of a project or an intervention can sometimes be unpredictable, incalculable or unseen. This is one of the fundamental arguments that question not only the cause/effect way of thinking about projects, but also the issues of certainty, control and prediction when explaining social facts or human change. It is also at the heart of the discussion on either attribution or contribution in monitoring and evaluation, evaluation and impact assessment.

Monitoring and evaluation approaches

The two approaches to monitoring and evaluation that will now be discussed offer a comprehensive approach to monitoring and evaluation as research and management functions from planning to evaluation. The results-based management approach is being used by large-scale and mid-scale organisations, and even governments, while outcome mapping is used by large-scale research organisations such as the International Development Research Centre (IDRC) in Canada, which has been its main developer. In the specific case of the UK, most projects and initiatives supported by local councils use the results-based management approach (see for example the Greenwich Strategy 2006–15). In Canada, the government, using the results-based management approach, has chosen user satisfaction as an indicator across all public services delivered (NEF, 2004).

The results-based management approach

The results-based management approach globally comprises three phases from planning to evaluation, each with specific tasks and tools (OECD, 2000):

- **Phase 1**: this corresponds to the strategic planning of a project or initiative in which clear and measurable objectives are defined, indicators to measure progress chosen and targets for indicators explicitly set. The main tool used is called, in some cases, the strategic results framework and it attempts to outline or summarise the main results to be achieved by a project or initiative (ideally with the participation of all stakeholders as suggested above) according to defined goals, sub-goals, strategic area(s) of support, period of time, type of results expected (outputs, outcomes, impacts) and indicators, depending upon the specific circumstances of a project or initiative.
- **Phase 2**: this comprises the performance measurement stage in which the monitoring system as such is set up; this consists of a data collection and data analysis strategy, including the use of qualitative or quantitative methods. The corresponding tools accompanying the monitoring system are the results-oriented annual reports, semestral reports and quarterly reports; these also depend upon the specific circumstances of the project or initiative. These tools are used for

reporting on the performance and progress of the results achieved according to the time stage.

- **Phase 3**: this is the results-based management stage itself in which all data collected are used as information for internal management, learning and decision making. Also, evaluation as a plan activity and research and management function are decided here.

The outcome mapping approach

The outcome mapping approach has a working logic similar to the results-based management approach. It defines itself as an assessment of outputs and outcomes rather than impacts. It further acknowledges the significant role of impact as the ultimate goal of a project or initiative but focuses on outcomes (Earl *et al.*, 2001). In its turn, a project's or initiative's outcomes are defined essentially as elements under the control of boundary partners (individuals, groups and organisations with whom the project or intervention interacts directly and with whom the project anticipates opportunities for influence). Outcome mapping sees projects or initiatives basically as a set of contributions to a process by providing access to new resources, ideas or opportunities within a specific period of time. In this context, accountability relates to outcomes, since it is what managers and bounded partners can manage, control and monitor. In a similar way to the results-based management approach, outcome mapping also comprises three phases that cover various specific tasks – from planning to evaluation – with the corresponding tools.

- **Phase 1**: this is the intentional design stage in which stakeholders define the vision (Why?), mission (How?), bounded partnerships (Who?), outcome challenges (What?), progress markers (When?), strategy maps and organisational practices for a project or initiative.
- **Phase 2**: this corresponds to the stage in which outcome(s) and the performance monitoring is set up. Thus, the monitoring priorities of a project or initiative are defined along with the three tools that contribute to the monitoring: outcomes journal (tool), strategy journal (tool) and performance journal (tool).
- **Phase 3**: this is the evaluation planning stage in which an evaluation plan is defined.

The differences between the results-based management framework and outcome mapping approaches

The main contrasting issues between these two approaches relate to the conceptualisation of results, attribution versus contribution, change and accountability versus learning. While the results-based management approach considers it possible to monitor and evaluate three main types of results – outputs, outcomes and impacts – the outcome mapping approach centres on the monitoring and evaluation of outputs and outcomes. Outcome mapping acknowledges the significance of impact(s) as the decisive goal of any project or initiative but focuses chiefly on outcomes (Earl et al., 2001).

The issue of attribution versus contribution to change is the second element that differs between the two approaches. The results-based management approach assumes that achievement of results (outcomes and impacts) can be attributed to an intervention, although not as a single or simple effect of an agent but the effect of a group of partners. As a result, this approach puts partnerships in a condition of attribution. Meanwhile, from the perspective of the outcome mapping approach, attribution of impact to an agent – in many instances, the financial one – contradicts the multiple endogenous contributions of all the other actors involved in a project or intervention as well as its future sustainability (Earl et al., 2001). Similarly, it implicitly demonstrates that power, control and decision making are in the hands of a few agents – the ones that provided the money, perhaps? Instead, the outcome mapping approach states that it is about contribution among boundary partners of a project or intervention and not just attribution to financial supporters.

Change is the next topic that differs between the two approaches. The results-based management approach defines results as a chain of cause-and-effect changes in which the three types of results take place. Outputs are defined as the completion of activities or services in a project or initiative, whereas outcomes are defined as the actual or intended mid-term changes. Impacts, meanwhile, are defined as the overall, sustainable and long-term changes brought about by a project or initiative. Outcome mapping, focusing mainly on outcomes, defines them as specific changes in behaviours, relationships, actions or activities of people, groups and organisations. The results-based management approach would consider that change, whether intended or unintended, positive or negative, could happen to a situation (wellbeing improvement), a stage (wellbeing in general) or human beings (wellbeing of end-users) as a consequence of a project or initiative, whereas the outcome mapping approach considers human change mainly as the fundamental element defining outcomes. In a wellbeing project or initiative using the outcome mapping approach, change would have occurred mainly when the individuals' behaviours, feelings, ideas, relations and actions around objective and subjective wellbeing had changed.

The last element of contrast between the two approaches is accountability versus learning. The results-based management approach addresses both learning and accountability, while the outcome mapping approach privileges learning and self-assessment over accountability.

Activity 4.1 Reflection

What wellbeing projects or initiatives are you aware of in your area? Gather documentation for two of these projects and identify their approach to monitoring and evaluation. If no approach is mentioned, what approach would you suggest would be appropriate?

WELLBEING CHARACTERISATION

Trying to clarify the category of wellbeing in order to discuss how to monitor and evaluate it in a project or initiative is a challenging task, as the literature on the subject is varied and complex. In this chapter, wellbeing is characterised according to two main meanings that, although related and overlapping, are the ones that the literature (Bourne, 2010; Cameron, 2006; Diener, 2009) shows will allow anybody eventually to make sense of the category of wellbeing when it comes to either monitoring or evaluating it. The two main definitions are wellbeing as a health phenomenon and wellbeing as life satisfaction or happiness.

Wellbeing as a health phenomenon

The most common and traditional characterisation of wellbeing is very closely associated with the notion of health as defined by the World Health Organization (WHO) in 1948 (Bourne, 2010; Cameron, 2006), in the sense that, if health is not merely the absence of disease, it is wellbeing – a state of complete physical, mental and social wellness. However, Bourne points out that, despite the efforts of WHO in making the definition of health as inclusive as possible from a bio-psychosocial perspective, health is still framed mainly from a biomedical perspective that constructs the notion of health as disease, material condition or dysfunction occurring in the body without consideration of any other element (Bourne, 2010). This means that, in many cases, health policies and projects when measuring wellbeing will mainly privilege the influence of biological or physical conditions and, nowadays, probably genetic conditions, at the expense of the influence of a set of interrelated aspects such as the bio-genetic, environmental, economic and sociological (Bourne, 2010; NEF, 2004).

Cameron *et al.* (2006), exploring notions of health and wellbeing in a project aimed at measuring aspects and determinants of health among professionals and community groups in the UK, came to the conclusion that the lack of clarity and holism of these notions could eventually create more problems than solutions for both health organisations and policy makers. This is the result of ignoring the specificities and qualitative aspects of notions of health and wellbeing carried out for a community as opposed to the ones formulated by policy makers and health organisations. In this particular case, even within the community itself, the characterisations of wellbeing varied according to age groups (younger and older), various ethnic groups, females and males, and rural and urban experiences (Cameron *et al.*, 2006), demonstrating quite well the interrelation of psychosocial factors, different cultural groups and individual aspects.

A bio-psychosocial approach to the understanding of wellbeing produces a broad model of health that is not exclusively medically oriented; it is a sense of positive health in contrast to negative health and the subjective dimensions of health (Cameron *et al.*, 2006). As Fisher *et al.* (2000) state, the category of wellbeing should certainly cover as many dimensions of one's being as possible. Thus, particularly when monitoring and evaluating wellbeing projects and initiatives, it is expected that the category of wellbeing will set up a comprehensive set of indicators related not only to physical health but also to crime, education, leisure, housing, social exclusion, the environment and subjective indicators (Bourne, 2010; Evans, 2005).

Wellbeing characterised as life satisfaction or happiness

Similar to the characterisation of wellbeing as a health issue, the category of wellbeing characterised as life satisfaction or happiness has some particularities that should be addressed when attempting to monitor or evaluate a wellbeing project or initiative. First, life satisfaction as an indicator of people's wellbeing has been related very much to the approach that measures economic growth or prosperity by calculating national and individual incomes. And, similarly to the case of wellbeing as a health category privileging bio-genetic aspects at the expense of others, in this case there is also some criticism of the economic approach that focuses mainly on material exchange and value at the expense of other complementary aspects such as social welfare and ecological sustainability (Bakshi, 2007; Diener, 2009; NEF, 2004). Thus, although income is a critical component when attempting to measure wellbeing, it cannot be the only indicator of economic growth, let alone happiness, since non-income indicators such as education, nutrition, immunisation, expenditure on public health and poverty reduction are also significant when monitoring and evaluating a wellbeing project or initiative (Bourne, 2010).

Second, wellbeing characterised as happiness highlights the most subjective aspects of health from a psychological perspective. Paraphrasing Diener's characterisation of SWB, this is the feeling an individual has about his or her life as something desirable, pleasant and good (Diener, 2009). Illustrating the hallmarks of his characterisation, Diener points out that this concept dwells within the experience of the individual, takes into account positive measures, and 'measures the global assessment of all aspects of a person's life' (p. 13). The area of SWB is flourishing in terms of research and development of more precise tools for its measurement. The New Economics Foundation's (NEF) model of wellbeing addresses, for example, two personal dimensions and a social context: life satisfaction, people's personal development and people's social wellbeing.

Therefore, when monitoring and evaluating a project or initiative related to wellbeing, it is important that the category of wellbeing is characterised as a multidimensional, multidisciplinary and multifaceted issue, as stated by Bourne (2010). Similarly, as he defines it, when monitoring and evaluating wellbeing, one should try to assess 'the overall health status of people, which includes access to and control over material resources, environmental and psychological conditions, and per capita consumption' (p. 20).

WHY, WHAT AND HOW TO MONITOR AND EVALUATE WELLBEING PROJECTS OR INITIATIVES

The fact that health, in its most ample meaning including wellbeing, is becoming 'everybody's business' – communities, individuals, health authorities, policy makers and researchers, as pointed out by Cameron *et al.* (2006) – provides the main rationale for wellbeing projects and initiatives to better monitor and evaluate it. The NEF's (2004) wellbeing manifesto states that social policies are the drivers of better thinking, better answers and better actions about wellbeing. If this is the case, a more accountable, research- and lesson-oriented monitoring and evaluation system for wellbeing projects and initiatives has the great responsibility of delivering a more effective and innovative health and wellbeing impact policy. It should be one that, as the NEF's manifesto adds, would allow us to assess a 'flourishing society, where citizens are happy, healthy, capable and engaged – in other words with high levels of wellbeing' (p. 2).

In terms of what to monitor and evaluate in wellbeing projects and initiatives, as discussed earlier, the basic international criteria used by multilateral organisations, governments and others in relation to any project are relevance, performance and success. Thus, these criteria should certainly provide the context as to what to essentially monitor and evaluate in a wellbeing project or initiative. In some cases, the category of performance is replaced by efficiency and effectiveness. Also, in some other cases the category of success is replaced by impact and sustainability. Both the results-based management and the outcome mapping approach to monitoring and evaluation include these criteria, although with variations.

The monitoring and evaluation of a wellbeing project or initiative can be carried out in seven and four main steps respectively. Most monitoring or participatory monitoring exercises as managerial and research functions of a wellbeing project or initiative can be carried out in the following seven steps, if the approach used is results-based management.

1. The stakeholders of a wellbeing project or initiative should agree on the type of results to be achieved along with the baseline from which they are starting (outputs/outcomes/impacts).

2. Next, they should also agree on the indicators. As was suggested, in a wellbeing project or initiative it is expected that the indicators will cover a range of aspects, from physical health to non-income activities such as nutrition and education.

3. With the stakeholders' consensus on the indicators, the next immediate steps are the consensus on and definition of a strategy for data collection and data analysis (see below for details of data collection and analysis under evaluation).

4. The following step should ideally be a reporting strategy outlining the content and frequency of reports (quarterly, six-monthly or annual) to be disseminated to the various stakeholders.

5. A list of roles and responsibilities of the monitoring activities is the next required step, so that the data collection and analysis is carried out with a certain research rigour and frequency.

6. A schedule of the main monitoring events of the wellbeing project or initiative is the next step. Most projects need training and capacity building in monitoring during the whole period when a project or initiative is being implemented.

7. The last step to be considered in the undertaking of the monitoring plan is the budget assigned to all the monitoring activities. The monitoring in some projects and initiatives is poor because many stakeholders do not allocate financial resources for monitoring activities.

If a project or initiative follows the outcome mapping approach, as opposed to the results-based management approach, the method for devising a monitoring plan mainly has to follow the outcome mapping approach. Evaluation of a project or initiative, on the other hand, can be carried out in the following four steps.

1. Translating the underpinning logic of the project or initiative into targeted evaluation questions using the criteria of relevance, performance and success.

2. Defining the methodology for data collection and data analysis. Covering as many quantitative and qualitative aspects of the project or initiative as possible should be a significant task. Although complementary, these methods respond to different aims and purposes. Triangulation, the blending and combination of the two approaches, is advisable although with some warning (Love *et al.*, 2005). Briefly, the following tools are used by each method:

   a. qualitative tools: interviews, focus groups, case studies, surveys with open-ended questions and, in some cases, content analysis of the social, economic and political context in which the project or initiative is taking place;

   b. quantitative methods: statistical analysis of all types, cost-benefit analysis, modelling and financial appraisal, and randomised control trials (Lazenbatt *et al.*, 2001).

3. Analysing the data collected with the corresponding synthesis and findings in relation to the evaluation questions.

4. Disseminating activity in which the findings, results and lessons learnt are presented to relevant audiences.

Activity 4.2 Reflection

What do you consider to be the advantages and disadvantages of the two approaches to monitoring and evaluation?

CONCLUSION

The purpose of presenting a framework for the monitoring and evaluation of wellbeing projects or initiatives responds to the national and international pressure for results, accountability and impact. Monitoring and evaluation as research and management functions can certainly contribute to systemising the experience of a project or initiative in a rigorous and effective way, so that all stakeholders can witness how people's lives improve on the one hand and, on the other, how policy makers take care of taxpayers' resources by deciding sensibly about which type of project and initiative makes sense in contrast to others.

Results-based management and outcome mapping are among the most interesting approaches currently available, not only to monitor and evaluate projects, but also as approaches to planning a project or an initiative from the very beginning. Although there are some basic differences between the two approaches regarding, for example, the conceptualisation of results – attribution versus contribution, and change and accountability versus learning – both approaches respond to the assumed logic that sees a set of linkages or chains among projects' or initiatives' resources (inputs), activities, results (outputs, outcomes and impacts), stakeholders and short-, mid- and long-term impact in relation to a situation or problem.

When setting up a monitoring and evaluation system for a wellbeing project or initiative, this has to be conceptualised as a multidimensional, multidisciplinary and multifaceted issue, as stated by Bourne (2010). Also, it has to be understood as the monitoring and evaluation of 'the overall health status of people, which includes access to and control over material resources, environmental and psychological conditions, and per capita consumption' (p. 20).

The clarification of results to be achieved, the definition of evaluation questions, the setting up of indicators, the setting up of methodological strategies including quantitative and qualitative research methods for collecting data, naming those responsible for monitoring and evaluation in a project, capacity building for monitoring and evaluation needs, and allocation of financial resources are among the most important tasks to be identified when devising monitoring and evaluation plans, according to the approach used. Once more, as the NEF's (2004) manifesto states, it is about monitoring and evaluating where we are in the process of building a 'flourishing society, where citizens are happy, healthy, capable and engaged – in other words with high levels of wellbeing' (p. 2).

Further reading and websites

The references below are the most comprehensive sources to provide additional information on the monitoring and evaluation approaches discussed in this chapter.

UNDP (2010) *Handbook on Monitoring and Evaluating for Results.* New York: Evaluation Office. Available electronically at **www.undp.org/evaluation/handbook**

Earl, S., Carden, F. and Smutylo, T. (2001) *Outcome Mapping: Building Learning and Reflection into Development Programmes.* IDRC. Available at **www.idrc.ca/en/ev-26586-201-1-DO_TOPIC.html**

Part 2: Psychological Aspects of Wellbeing

Chapter 5

Psychoneuroimmunology and Wellbeing

Christine Stacey

Learning outcomes

In this chapter you will learn:

- how psychoneuroimmunology relates to wellbeing;

- to understand that wellbeing requires knowledge of the relationship between the primitive brain and physiological responses;

- to be aware of how everything we do over any 24 hour time period exerts influence on our immune system.

This chapter focuses on how emotion affects immunity, which in turn affects bodily function and wellbeing. Psychoneuroimmunology provides the link between Activities of Daily Living (ADL) and the body's response through the immune system encompassing the micro-wellbeing of individuals, while also acknowledging that individual wellbeing cannot be considered in isolation from the macro determinants of wellbeing.

INTRODUCTION

That we remain alive, according to Guyton and Hall (2006), is beyond our control in that hunger drives us to eat, fear to seek refuge, cold warmth and other primitive drivers to reproduction. While there is no doubt that our primitive brain, particularly the limbic system, exerts huge influence over behaviour, this very simplistic definition fails to take into account the power of the human mind or the role of emotion in determining wellbeing. Although Guyton and Hall consider that the human functions as an automaton, Damasio (2000) argues that subjective irrational emotion is increasingly implicated in somatoform disease, although direct provenance is difficult to establish. Nevertheless, the human body functions optimally within a narrow chemical variation, striving to maintain a level of homeostasis that allows normal functionality. When this cannot be achieved chaos ensues, which means effectively that the chemicals that drive us are out of control, with resulting ill health (Martinez-Lavin et al., 2008). Without homeostasis we not only suffer myriad illnesses from minor malfunctions to major organ or system disruption, but also remove the human body's innate ability to heal (Taniguchi et al., 2009).

THE BACKGROUND TO PSYCHONEUROIMMUNOLOGY

Research in the relationship between the brain and immune systems has been taking place since the 1920s. Although in the 1950s there was passing interest in the theory that stress may influence how the immune system functions in relationship to infectious disease, it was not until the 1970s, when links between the brain and immune system were identified, that specific research was initiated (Ader, 2001). The discovery of signalling neuropeptides in the 1980s (Pert et al., 1985) triggered the discipline of psychoneuroimmunology (PNI). Finding the overt connection between this discovery and that lymphocytes have both receptors and a secretory capability for these signals (Pert et al., 1998) has developed a gradual shift in the approach to management of health and disease. As research into the role of the immune system advanced, alongside understanding how these neuropeptides including neurotransmitters, hormones, cytokines and growth factors were also related (Pert et al., 1998), the significance of the role of mind–body– health relationships increased. However, despite this evidence, the biomedical approach continues to dominate.

THE PHYSIOLOGY OF PSYCHONEUROIMMUNOLOGY

Homeostasis is defined by Guyton and Hall (2006) as the maintenance of the nearly constant condition of the internal environment, and it is this balance of internal mechanisms that holds the key to PNI. However, as our external environment has changed faster than the human body has adapted, disruption is common. Such influences range from our external environment, including where and how we live and our mobilisation – using mechanical transport instead of walking alters the environment by changing the construct of the air we breathe – to what and how we eat. Within this is encapsulated society and how we relate to each other both in intimate and not-so-intimate relationships. Adaptation has provided human beings with a huge cortex allowing superior cognitive functioning, although the much smaller primitive brain continues to be the driving force of our most basic needs. Therefore, the body constantly seeks homeostasis with the complex intertwined controls of the nervous, endocrine and immune systems within the daily conflict of existence in the twenty-first century.

The physiology of emotion

The limbic system refers to the entire neuronal circuitry that controls emotional behaviour and motivational drives, including the structures of the diencephalon; the thalamus, hypothalamus, hippocampus and amygdala.

- The thalamus is responsible for the exchange of sensory information between receptors and the brain, excluding smell.
- The hypothalamus is responsible for responsive communication between the organs and visceral structures, including sexual stimuli, appetite and pain.
- The hippocampus is implicated in memory.
- The amygdala is concerned with perception and processing of emotion and memory.

These organs are linked by an arch consisting of assorted neural tracts in direct communication with the cerebral cortex. The cortex is considered to be the executive suite of the nervous system responsible for motivation, cognition, perception, communication, understanding, appreciation and the initiation of voluntary movement. No area of the brain works alone, therefore all conscious or responsive behaviour involves the cortex in some way. Stimulation of the limbic system, particularly where intense emotion is concerned, also results in extreme cerebral excitability that can manifest itself, for instance, as 'rage'. When we 'feel' an emotion the limbic system transforms it into the chemical cascade that instantaneously prepares the body for fight or flight, or a sexual interaction that occurs without having to be consciously 'switched on'. It is an autonomic nervous system response trigged by emotion.

Activity 5.1 Emotion and body systems

This activity enables you to consider how emotion directly affects physiology.

1. Sit quietly and think about an incident that distressed you – how do you feel? Has your pulse rate risen? Are you breathing more quickly? Do you feel slightly nauseous?
2. Repeat but think of something that made you feel happy and then reflect on how your body is responding? Do you notice any changes?

Physiologically, if you are walking down a dark street and you hear footfalls behind you, you 'feel' fear.

- Heart and respiratory rates increase (transport of nutrients and oxygen).
- Blood pressure rises.
- Increased blood flow to muscles and strength (preparation to run or fight).
- Decreased blood flow to gastrointestinal and renal systems (do not need to digest or urinate).
- Increased cellular metabolism (including the immune system as it prepares for body damage).
- Increased glycolysis and blood sugar concentration (energy for fight or flight).
- Increased mental agility (decision to fight or run).

(Guyton and Hall, 2006)

This state of extreme arousal, the result of activation of the hypothalamic-pituitary-adrenal (HPA) axis by strong emotion, can only be maintained for minutes. However, if the arousal continues, this is followed immediately by cortical secretion of cortisol.

Smell

Wellbeing is influenced by our environment. For example, happy feelings are often associated with odours, such as the smell of newly mown grass or ozone, which evoke thoughts of summer, and these happy feelings trigger endorphins. Conversely, unpleasant smells trigger the HPA axis to increase cortisol secretion. The piriform lobe, sited deep in the diencephalon in the medial aspect of the temporal lobes, collects afferent stimuli from sensory neurons in the nasal septi, giving consciousness of odour (Guyton and Hall, 2006). Although evolution has resulted in olfaction no longer being a primary sense for safety in extreme conditions, the phrase 'smell fear' is not unusual. For instance, as Trimble (2010) remarks when reflecting on medical students waiting to take their practical examinations, 'the rank stench of fear is easily identifiable' (p. 151), resulting from either HPA activation and associated physiological changes or increased circulating cortisol. In twenty-first-century man the olfactory bulbs and tracts have greatly reduced, with the olfactory cortex the only portion still sufficiently developed to receive smell in humans. As important as smell is to wellbeing, some smell can be unconscious and there is speculation that our choice of mate is connected with pheromones, although none have been identified in humans so far. There is also evidence that smell is associated in particular with memory retrieval. This concept has been used to improve the wellbeing of elderly people as smell is often associated with the 'where' memory-triggering memory cues (Ferrarini et al., 2010).

Circadian rhythm

Continuing with the concept of synergy with the world in which we live, homeostasis is controlled to some extent by the 24 hour circadian internal clock. As evening or darkness approaches there is a concomitant fall in body temperature and an increase in melatonin secretion preparing the body for sleep, the onset of which is accompanied by an increase in lactotrope prolactin from the pituitary and growth hormone from the hypothalamus (Hastings et al., 2003). During sleep, cortisol reaches its lowest ebb at about 3.00 a.m., then gradually rises to its peak on awakening due to the secretion of adrenocorticotropic hormone (ACTH), which helps activate awakening response with light-induced signals (Bryant et al., 2004). Cortisol levels increase for approximately two hours after waking to help stimulate ADL, after which they gradually fall throughout the day. During sleep the anabolic functions of growth and repair occur, whereas daytime activity is catabolic to allow interaction with ADL. However, if cortisol levels remain high, this can cause difficulty in both sleeping and staying asleep. Sleep is a necessity for recharging and revitalising the immune system, with research demonstrating that lack of sleep is associated with a reduction in immune response, including fewer circulating and less active Natural Killer (NK) cells, T cells and monocyte function (Irwin, 2002). Crucially, twenty-first-century life in the developed world continues regardless of time of day or night, resulting in social and commercial pressure for physical and mental activity regardless of where it is in any 24 hour cycle. Consider, for instance, how travelling across time zones disrupts homeostasis and the sleep/wake cycle or circadian rhythm and, therefore, its impact on the aetiology of wellbeing (Hastings *et al.*).

Light

Circadian rhythm homeostasis is reliant on the external stimulus of light and internal stimuli including the secretion of melatonin from the pineal gland and cortisol levels. The role and purpose of the pineal gland has intrigued researchers for many years and has been considered the 'seat of the soul', responsible for 'enhancing sex', 'promoting sleep', 'enhancing mood', and it is even thought to 'enhance longevity' and is implicated in the regulation of our sex lives (Guyton and Hall, 2006, p. 1009). The most important aspect is that this gland is controlled by the amount of light seen by the eyes in any 24 hour period. These light signals are transported to the suprachiasmal nucleus of the hypothalamus, which processes the length of day and night via the retina or photoreceptors (which are still functional in the blind), then signals to the pineal gland to activate secretion of melatonin (Guyton and Hall), and is implicated in the establishment of sleeping patterns in babies (Peirano *et al.*, 2003). Some tumours associated with the pineal gland secrete excessive quantities of pineal hormones, while others exert external pressure, reducing hormonal section (Guyton and Hall). Both types of tumour result in gonadal or hypergonadal dysfunction, indicating a role for the pineal gland in sexual function.

The role of light and how our physiology responds to it is further explored by Hastings *et al.* who concluded that the relationship between light and sleep is implicated in the response to disease and to medications for disease. There is some indication that melatonin disruption may be implicated in an increase in breast cancer and melanoma (Kvaskoff and Weinstein, 2010). Studies also indicate that disruption of the sleep–wake cycle predisposes to depression and Seasonal Affective Disorder (SAD) (Francis *et al.*, 2008), and there is evidence that poor sleepers find it harder to manage minor life stressors (Morin *et al.*, 2003).

Sleep

Normal sleep consists of two stages, Rapid Eye Movement (REM) and non-Rapid Eye Movement (nREM) or Slow Wave Sleep (SWS). nREM is 75 per cent of our sleep and consists of transition, total and deep delta wave sleep. REM is 25 per cent of our sleep and consists of tonic and phasic components during which the heart rate and respiration slow, routine physiological functions such as digestion decrease (Rosenwasser, 2009) and nonessential neurotransmitter activity ceases (Bryant *et al.*,

2004). Lack of sleep or insomnia is often associated with stress, anxiety and depression (Spoormaker and Bout, 2005), which themselves foster elevation of cortisol levels, therefore further disrupting the circadian rhythm (Buckley and Schatzberg, 2005). Total prevalence of insomnia is 10–30 per cent of the population (Spoormaker and Bout, 2005), and insomnia is higher in women over 45, particularly in those with a psychiatric history, low socio-economic status, chronic work stress, caregiver strain, hostility or who are socially isolated, with long-term sleep disruption implicated in the disruption of ADL, lack of concentration and significant accident mortality (Bryant et al., 2004).

Melatonin enhances cytokine production, including interleukins and other lymphokines implicated in cellular messaging that coordinates and stimulates lymphocyte activity (Glover et al., 2005). These crucial peptides function as autocrine, paracrine or endocrine hormones (Guyton and Hall, 2006), therefore difficulty in getting to sleep or remaining asleep may compromise the body's ability to fight bacterial and viral disease, as well as the body's ability to control the Human Immunodeficiency Virus (HIV) and cancer (Glover et al., 2005). Without rest, NK activity is at its lowest, leaving the body critically weakened and at risk from opportunistic as well as invading pathogens (Hui et al., 2007). Additionally there is some evidence suggesting that continual nocturnal activation of these neurotransmitters results in the lack of energy and lethargy that is invariably a feature of sleep deprivation and most illnesses (Rosenwasser, 2009). Furthermore, without rest memory is impaired, poor daytime motor coordination is common, low mood persists until exhaustion results and this is a cause for concern when ADL can no longer be maintained (Morikawa et al., 2005; Shakhar et al., 2007).

The immune system

The prime directive of the immune system is to protect its host body from harm and it comprises a highly complex and interactive combination of lymphatic vessels, organs and secretions that protect and support homeostasis. Harm can be external from invading pathogens, parasites or when structural integrity is compromised, or protection from internal harm when the immune system recognises cellular degeneration in order to protect against cancer (Westermann and Exton, 1999). The immune system consists of cellular and humoral responses. The former focuses on non-specific pathogens and inflammation including T lymphocyte cells (T cells), while humoral response focuses more on particular diseases and atopic reactions and involves B lymphocyte cells (B cells) and antibodies (Goldsby et al., 2002).

There are more than one type of T and B cells and both are produced in bone marrow. T cells then migrate to the outer cortex of the thymus gland where they mature and are programmed to identify their host's own proteins (T cell – T = thymus) and, while some migrate to lodge in lymphoid organs, many remain patrolling in the circulation (Goldsby *et al.*). B cells mature within the marrow from the preprocessing bursa of Faricius (B = bursa) and, once mature, they also migrate to lodge in organs of the lymphatic system, although in different parts of the body (Goldsby *et al.*). The main subsets of T cells are the T Helper (CD4) and the T cytotoxic (CD8) or NK cells (Goldsby *et al.*). After a CD4 T cell recognises and interacts with a major histocompatibility complex (MHC) it becomes an effector cell that secretes cytokines that play a major role in the proliferation of B cells, CD8 T cells and macrophages. Macrophages travel to sites under all epithelial and lymphoid tissue and non-lymphoid organs and recognise invading pathogens which they destroy through phagocytic activity. Tumour Necrosing Factor (TNF-α) is a cytokine secreted by activated macrophages and, alongside NK cells, it is implicated in the early recognition and destruction of cancerous cells. There is evidence suggesting that emotion exerts an effect on the circulating numbers of NK cells and on the secretion of TNF-α (Goldsby *et al.*). However, it is during sleep that the cells of the immune system are produced and activated, with NK cells interacting with dendritic cells for optimum cellular activation (Hui *et al.* 2007).

MIND–BODY MEDICINE

PNI teaches us that an imbalance in the flow of information between mind and body via neuropeptides and the resultant loss of physiological homeostasis results in chronic disease affecting individual wellbeing. The hypothalamus responds to perceived stress with a chain reaction of events compromising homeostasis, but it is particularly the secretion of excessive cortisol that is implicated in immune disruption as cortisol disrupts circadian rhythm (Ranjit *et al.*, 2005), therefore disrupting sleep without which there is decreased anabolic activity, resulting in illness and disease.

Irritable bowel disease

Irritable Bowel Disease (IBD) is an increasingly common chronic functional disorder of the lower bowel with unknown aetiology, but it is associated with significant morbidity. Pain, anxiety, psychosocial stress and depression are often co-morbidities, although which initiates which remains under debate. Much of the literature supports wellbeing and lifestyle changes, particularly establishing quality of life, as imperative for any meaningful improvement in symptoms (Rapps *et al.*, 2008). In PNI terms, a persistent low-grade inflammatory response with increased numbers of subsets of T cells including CD3+, CD4+ and CD25+ are implicated in creating symptoms (Andoh *et al.*, 2007). Additionally, proinflammatory cytokines Il-6 and TNF-α have been identified in the gut of IBD sufferers (Liebregts *et al.*, 2007). Increased mast cell activity in the colonic mucosa, releasing tryptase and activating protease-activated receptor-2 in nerves, may also predispose to the cycles of spasm and relaxation that cause the abdominal cramping (Kawabata *et al.*, 2008). Sleep disruption is usual, although probably secondary to anxiety, as IBD symptoms tend to resolve at night. However, as sleep disruption enhances inflammatory responses while reducing positive immune cellular activity, it can be extrapolated that interventions that foster positive mood may favourably affect the development and maintenance of dysregulated neuroimmune and endocrine systems underlying conditions such as IBD.

Case study 5.1 Cancer and HIV

The word 'cancer' and the diagnosis of cancer or HIV triggers an HPA response. Disruption of emotional wellbeing affects physical wellbeing, which is of particular significance with a diagnosis of cancer as it is imperative that there are sufficient numbers of both circulating and sufficiently active NK cells. Although researching cancer is fraught with difficulties, an increasing body of evidence identifies the role of emotion in survival. For instance, DeBrabander and Gerits (1999) established that both acute and chronic stress unassociated with the diagnosis were predictors of relapse. More recently, Groenvold *et al.* (2007) established that emotional wellbeing is linked to overall increased survival rate in breast cancer. Studies into reducing circulating cortisol using therapies such as massage indicate evidence to support the use of such therapies within cancer and palliative care (Hernandez-Reif *et al.*, 2004). Finally, Witek-Janusek *et al.* (2008) found that providing emotional support for women newly diagnosed with breast cancer improved their quality of life, therefore improving their immune function. With regard to HIV, any intervention whether physical, emotional or psychosocial that supports the immune system, maintaining circulating mature and active T and NK cells, must have a positive outcome.

EMOTIONAL HEALTH AND WELLBEING

Within the concept of emotion disrupting the immune system and affecting wellbeing, there are multiple applications and this section will only touch briefly on some of the more common. Once it is accepted that anything and everything we do independently influences immune function, and that optimism predicts better psychological adjustment to stress, it is clear that the ways in which we as individuals manage our ADL will affect our wellbeing. For instance, research indicates that environmental change including moving home and/or job triggers the HPA axis. Studies on happiness have concluded that security is essential, which may be economic (and account for the rise in happiness as poor communities and societies get richer), but also includes security of relationships, work and freedom. Offer *et al.* (2010) argue comprehensively that obesity is a result of market liberalism forces that engender fear of starvation or economic insecurity, as in a recession, resulting in the subsequent natural desire to eat and store food; in other words, the anxiety of recession causes obesity.

Many individuals live in isolation, with significant morbidity associated with old age. Pinquart and Sorensen (2001) investigated social interventions, Cattan *et al.* (2005) looked at social isolation and NICE (2008) advocated that walking and physical exercise programmes promoted wellbeing. Jakobsson *et al.* (2010) demonstrated that elderly individuals with a social network are therefore less lonely, and were therefore also less likely to be depressed, have significant lower morbidity and therefore less interaction with health services; loneliness was considered to be the significant factor. From the PNI perspective, reducing isolation encourages individuals to be socially interactive, which also has the effect of maintaining mobility, exposing them to natural light, and encouraging nocturnal sleep when the anabolic processes take place. Jakobsson *et al.* (2010) also concluded that individuals who had others in their social environment that they trusted directly correlated with reduced depression and morbidity.

Anyone living with chronic disease, particularly if this includes chronic pain, is likely to experience depression, anxiety and sleep disorders, further exacerbating physical symptoms (Irwin *et al.*, 2008). In Chronic Fatigue Syndrome (CFS), improving NK function has been shown to reduce fatigue (Meeus *et al.*, 2009), and an increased prevalence of emotive coping in CFS patients is associated with reduced fatigue, pain severity and overall disability.

CONCLUSION

Anxiety, depression, isolation, sadness, emotional and physical pain, lack of trust and other common co-morbidities affect sleep, thereby disrupting our circadian rhythms, compounding our emotional interface with homeostasis, interfering with our immune system's ability to keep us free from harm and destabilising our wellbeing. Wellbeing therefore needs to be tackled holistically by individuals and health and social care professionals from the dimension of understanding what each individual needs to function successfully; that is, the required balance between the basic needs of sleep, trust, caring and exposure to light in order to enhance wellbeing and reduce morbidity.

Further reading

Daruna, J.H. (2004) *Introduction to Psychoneuroimmunology*. London: Elsevier
A useful basic text that explains the discipline.

Pert, C.B. (1999) *Molecules of Emotion*. London: Simon and Schuster
Provides an understanding of the relationships between wellbeing and the immune system.

Chapter 6

Psychological Aspects of Wellbeing

Ben Bruneau

Learning outcomes

In this chapter you will learn how to:

- identify the psychological components that exist within the concepts of health and wellbeing;

- examine the various psychological issues that may affect people's health and wellbeing;

- assess people's psychological deficits with regard to their health and wellbeing;

- evaluate the approaches to be used to remedy these deficits.

INTRODUCTION

This chapter discusses the psychological aspects relevant to wellbeing. Using a physiopsychosocial model, it initially demonstrates the relationship between health and wellbeing. It then identifies how wellbeing is achievable through a balanced state of mind. Within that approach it considers behavioural, emotional and cognitive attributes, the set of psychological factors which contribute to wellbeing.

WELLBEING AND HEALTH

Wellbeing is almost always discussed in relation to health (see, for example, Kiefer, 2008). Health is, therefore, first considered. It is a concept and as such is subject to individual and group interpretation. Most people and nations have some common idea of what health is but its exact definition is far from being universally agreed. Various authorities see the present situation as acceptable since what is known as health seems to vary from country to country and from one time period to another. Generally, the definition is adaptable. Such an adaptation is found in the World Health Organization's (WHO) first attempt at defining health in 1946 and its subsequent, newer definition in 1984 and in the Ottawa Charter for Health Promotion (WHO, 1986). Today, however, the definition that was formalised by WHO in 1946, that health is a state in which the individual does not experience disease but enjoys a 'complete state of physical, social and mental wellbeing', remains firm and is the most commonly quoted and generally acceptable definition (Üstün and Jakob, 2005). This is in spite of the newer definition that suggests that health is the ability to realise aspirations, satisfy needs and change or cope with the environment (WHO, 1984). Health ultimately points to a link between a positive physical, psychological and social state (see Figure 6.1). Within that state the concept of wellbeing is implied. Therefore, wellbeing, in the context of health, is simply interpreted as the state of being well and not having any type of complaints, be they physical, psychological or sociological.

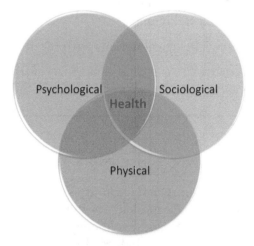

Figure 6.1 The basic components relevant within the concept of health

Further, general references to health are commonly focused around having good physical health. Huppert and Bayliss (2004) argue that whenever health is investigated it almost invariably has to do with physical health problems rather than with other aspects, such as vitality and physical thriving, that are known to play a part in wellbeing.

While wellbeing itself is not defined by WHO (1946), it is viewed as a state of happiness and satisfaction with life (Kahneman *et al.*,1999), having a focus on a sound psychological state. It too points to the absence of complaints and disease, and also refers to the satisfaction aspect suggested by the WHO's 1984 revised definition of health. However, Schickler (2005), for example, suggests that being well, in the sense of not having a disease, does not constitute wellbeing. Wellbeing is more than that. It is generally regarded as to do with how the individual achieves his or her potential and undertakes what he or she wants to undertake on account of personal vitality and energy. Wellbeing is thus referred to as psychological wellbeing, for it is argued to be about goals, hopes and aspirations, all aspects that are seated in the mind. In this understanding, Kiefer (2008) stipulates a set of components when referring to wellbeing. These components are the individual characteristics of people, which refer to people's ability to function on their own and to their physical and mental health; their physical and living environment factors; their social and socioeconomic factors; the subjective satisfaction of their quality of life; psychological health; their outside activities and life changes; and the care they receive or anticipate. Ultimately, those components have their origin in the physical, psychological and sociological areas (see Figure 6.2), the same three components found in the health concept.

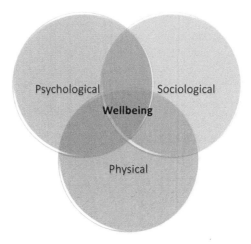

Figure 6.2 The basic components that are relevant within the concept of wellbeing

Psychological wellbeing is usually considered to have two distinct types: hedonic wellbeing and eudemonic wellbeing (see also Chapter 3). Hedonic wellbeing focuses on an individual's feeling of continuum with life (Diener *et al.*, 2002; Kahneman *et al.*, 1999). It refers to short-term pleasures such as the type elicited by the senses. It is concerned with feelings of contentment with life. Eudemonic wellbeing emphasises the individual's meaningful engagement in life and their self-realisation (Ryan and Reci, 2001; Ryff and Singer, 2008). It is concerned with the sustainability of wellbeing associated with an individual's utilisation of their strengths, the fostering of their relationships and working towards socially desirable goals. Ryff (1989b) proposes a widely accepted model of behaviour for eudemonic wellbeing, consisting of six dimensions (see Table 6.1).

The Ryff Scale

Aspects measured: The respondent's:

1. Autonomy:

    Capacity to be self-determining and independent

2. Environmental mastery:

    Capacity to effectively manage everyday life and create a surrounding context that fits with personal needs and values

3. Personal growth:

    Sense of continuing growth and self-realisation

4. Positive relations with others:

    Good-quality relationships with others

5. Purpose in life:

    Sense that life is purposeful and meaningful

6. Self-acceptance:

    Having positive regard for one's self and one's past life

Table 6.1 The six dimensions measured by the Ryff Scale

The initial approach, therefore, when considering health and wellbeing, is that these two terms and the concepts they represent are, in the very least, interrelated by the stance they take: that of being well in common domains. This is indeed confirmed by Schickler (2005), and it is because of this interrelationship that these terms are also often used interchangeably. But this would not be a true representation of the two concepts or states. Their further consideration suggests that they can be seen as distinct, different one from the other. Schickler, for instance, goes on to demonstrate that although there is a clear interrelationship between the two states, wellbeing has a wider meaning than health, that it can exist in the absence of health and that health itself can also occur without wellbeing. Schickler argues the point made by Gallie (1956), who suggests that although on the surface health and wellbeing cover many common attributes at the same time, their meanings are different and, most importantly, these meanings remain contested. In spite of all this, there has been a distinct attempt in the last 30 years to better understand the concepts (see Beattie *et al.*, 1993; Helman, 1994; Kleiman, 1988; Milburn, 1996; Stainton Rogers, 1991) and the relevant part they occupy in professional repertoires.

The concepts convey positive states that professionals would like individuals and groups of individuals to achieve. There is now a generally accepted view that the two concepts can exist separately but that they can also coexist (Schickler, 2005). Importantly, however, psychological entities are seen to be an integral part of the concepts. Mental wellbeing is mentioned in the WHO (1946) definition of health. The presence of mental wellbeing in health, the positive emotion conveyed by states of happiness, and the satisfaction with life, a positive cognitive perception in wellbeing, amount to the presence of psychological wellbeing.

The contribution of psychology to health and wellbeing suggests that people are generally viewed as having an influence on the state they experience and it would seem that in the consideration of their attitudes a characteristic such as their perceived behavioural control has also a crucial part to play. This psychological aspect deserves further consideration.

PSYCHOLOGY AND WELLBEING

Psychology, literally translated from the Ancient Greek as 'the study of the mind', does more than just investigate the processes of the mind. It also considers human behaviour, which, although this can be considered as distinct and separate from the activities of the mind, is often understood to be the result of mental processes. Eventually, psychology finds itself studying people's behaviour, thinking and, inevitably, their affect or emotions, an aspect that clearly becomes apparent when human nature is placed under scrutiny. These aspects can be encapsulated within the acronym BET – B for behaviour, E for emotions, T for thinking – which is often referred to, and commonly understood, as cognition. Thus, psychology sets out to observe and report on what people do under certain circumstances, what their expressed and unexpressed feelings might be under various conditions, and their thoughts and learning processes that might be involved in and have an impact on their behaviour and feelings. This type of approach often yields results suggesting that these three aspects are often related and can be a useful consideration in the area of health and wellbeing (Bruneau, 2009).

When individual health is considered, the person's behaviour, feelings and thoughts are all relevant and are seen to have a distinct influence on the eventual healthiness and wellness of the person. A mental (therefore psychological) aspect is often seen as relevant. This is clearly seen when individuals, and later groups, are examined for their contribution to their health and wellbeing. Extensive work has been done in the field of attitudes and how these attitudes play a role in how people feel, and the state they find themselves in. Attitudes are argued to have three components (see, for example, Aronson *et al.*, 2005; Hogg and Vaughan, 2005; Morrison and Bennett, 2006), known as ABC: an affective (A) component, dealing with the feelings attached to an object; a behavioural (B) component, expressed in the predisposition of acting towards an object in a certain way; and a cognitive (C) component, which refers to the beliefs about the object. The existence of an attitude can be illustrated in the following expression about an object: 'Oliver likes to eat organic food'. 'Likes' is the affect part that enables Oliver to deal with the object, organic food; 'eat' is to do with the behaviour he shows towards that object – he eats organic food; and 'organic' suggests a belief that Oliver has for such a type of food. Perhaps he thinks such food is better for him than other types of food (for example, chemically aided food or genetically modified food). Some psychologists believe that attitudes have a part to play in the state of health and the state of wellbeing. Fishbein and Ajzen (1975), for example, use an attitude variable in the explanation of people's actions. In their Theory of Reasoned Action (TRA), the influence of an attitude in behaviour is depicted as related to the other elements of the theory. Likewise, when positing his Theory of Planned Behaviour (TPB), an extension of TRA, Ajzen (1991) argues for an element of attitude within that theory. Both TRA and TPB postulate that individuals are rational in considering their actions and the implications of their actions. Figures 6.3 and 6.4 display the specific elements of the two theories. TPB is particularly seen as providing more clarity on the individual as a rational being when it introduces the variable of perceived behavioural control. Perceived behavioural control is a person's perception on how easily he or she can carry out an action.

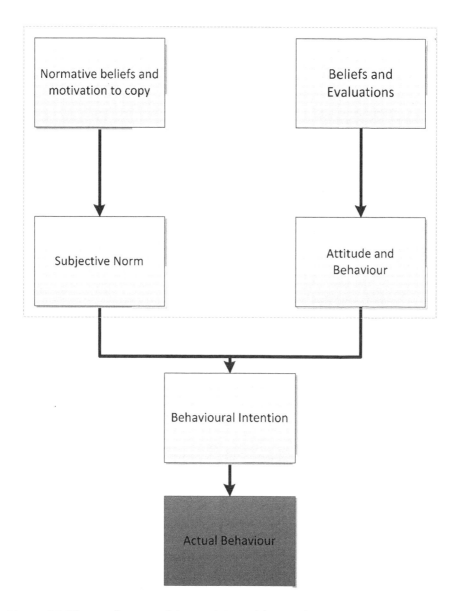

Figure 6.3 Theory of Reasoned Action (adapted from Fishbein and Ajzen, 1975)

Therefore, people are generally viewed as having some influence on the state they experience and it would seem that, in the consideration of their attitudes, a characteristic such as their perceived behavioural control also has a crucial part to play. In a definition of wellbeing, Kiefer (2008) argues that the concept is synonymous with happiness and with health, among other attributes. Weston and Hughes (1999) postulate

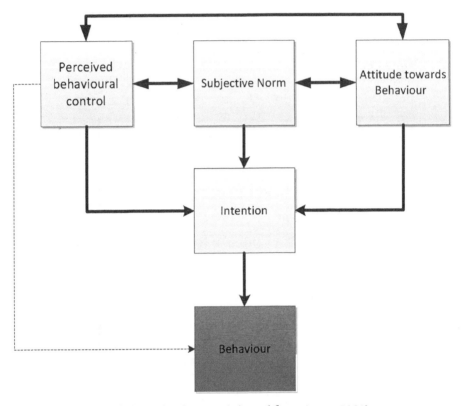

Figure 6.4 Theory of Planned Behaviour (adapted from Ajzen, 1991)

that happiness or unhappiness cannot be inferred on the basis of objective circumstances alone and that personal interpretation of circumstances is viewed as crucial in the inference. Further, Huppert and Bayliss (2004) emphasise that most researchers focus on the psychological rather than the physical and social states when they investigate wellbeing. Thus, personal attributes are required. One of these attributes is control, more precisely a person's ability to control his or her environment. Shapiro *et al.* (1996) argue that losing control is one of life's greatest fears, and that the individual therefore is always striving to keep that control.

Other theories have considered what role particular aspects of the mind play in health and wellbeing. One example is the theory of personality and the role personality types may play in keeping an individual healthy (see, for example, Ryckman, 2004), and the theory of self-efficacy (Bandura, 1977), which strongly places the onus on the individual's own ability to keep healthy. These theories are all relevant to the understanding of health and wellbeing.

PSYCHOLOGICAL INTERVENTIONS IN HEALTH AND WELLBEING

The multifaceted nature of wellbeing suggests that in order to experience wellbeing, a balance must be established among the facets. In order to achieve such equilibrium, an individual is required to be vigilant for problems that may arise with any of the facets. That vigilance becomes the focus of the health practitioner. In looking at what has to be done to maintain, promote or restore wellbeing, an assessment of wellbeing has to be made and, once the wellbeing state is known, interventions can then take place.

The assessment of problems pertaining to wellbeing

Wellbeing is undoubtedly a dynamic concept, consisting of a large number of components. As discussed earlier, these components span subjective, environmental, psychological and health-related behaviour dimensions. They include individual characteristics of people, social, living environment, socioeconomic and physical environment factors, personal autonomy, subjective satisfaction, psychological health, activities, life changes and care (Kiefer, 2008). They also amount to a consideration of how people feel (for example, there is a focus on people's positive affect, negative affect and life satisfaction) and how well people perceive aspects of their functioning (for example, the perceived amount of control they feel they have of their lives, the feeling of whether what they do is worthwhile, and whether they have good relationships with others). Abbott *et al.* (2006) demonstrate that this consideration can ultimately lead to the assessment of people's psychological wellbeing. The multifaceted concept of psychological wellbeing should therefore be surveyed by measures able to assess most, if not all, of the concept's components. One particular measure with three versions, Ryff's Scales of Psychological Wellbeing (PWB) (Ryff, 1989), has been designed to achieve this purpose.

The Ryff PWBs set out to measure psychological wellbeing covering the components discussed in this chapter but they are based on a eudemonic perspective rather than the hedonic perspective of subjective wellbeing. The hedonic perspective is not measured as it is generally understood as being fleeting and inconsistent in nature and as such is not a stable, and therefore not a reliable, indication of wellbeing. Two of the three scales (the long form, consisting of 84 questions, and the medium form, with 54 questions) have been shown to be valid and reliable in many studies since their inception in 1989 (see, for example, Bauer and McAdams, 2004; Cheng and Chang, 2005; Fava *et al.*, 2003; Lindfords *et al.*, 2006; Ruini and Fava, 2009; Ryff and Singer, 2008). The third scale (a short form of 18 questions) is not recommended as it is statistically unreliable (personal correspondence with Carol Ryff, author of the scales, 2010). In order to show the usefulness of the Ryff PWBs in the context of health and wellbeing, the long form is referred to as an illustration. The form consists of a series of statements reflecting the six areas (or dimensions) that ultimately make up psychological wellbeing.

Table 6.2 shows an extract from the 84-item scale (the long version) giving example statements for each of the categories of wellbeing measured by the Ryff scale. Respondents rate the statements on a scale of 1 to 6, with 1 indicating strong disagreement and 6 indicating strong agreement with a particular statement. Responses are totalled for each of the six categories. During analysis, about half of the responses, which are indicated on the master copy of the scale, are reverse-scored. For each category, a high score indicates that the respondent has a mastery of that area in their life. Conversely, a low score in a category shows that the respondent is struggling in that particular area. The score is interpreted and explained in the following way for each of the dimensions (see, for example, Seifert, 2005.

Autonomy

A high score in autonomy indicates that the respondent is self-determined and independent, while a low score suggests that the respondent is concerned about others' expectations and evaluations.

Environmental mastery

A high score in environmental mastery suggests the respondent has a sense of mastery and competence in managing the environment, while a low score shows that the respondent has difficulty managing everyday affairs.

Personal growth

A high score in personal growth indicates that an individual has a feeling of continued development, while a low score conveys an individual's sense of personal stagnation.

Positive relations with others

A high score in the positive relations with others dimension indicates the individual has warm, satisfying and trusting relationships with

The Ryff Scale

To the respondent: For each of the following six items concerned with wellbeing a statement is made. Please respond to a statement by choosing one number, using the response choices listed just below

1 = strongly disagree, 2 = disagree, 3 = Disagree a little, 4 = agree a little,

5 = agree, 6 = strongly agree

1	*Autonomy:*
	I have confidence in my opinions, even if they are contrary to the general consensus
	1 2 3 4 5 6
2	*Environmental mastery:*
	In general, I feel I am in charge of the situation in which I live
	1 2 3 4 5 6
3	*Personal growth:*
	I think it is important to have new experiences that challenge how you think about yourself and the world
	1 2 3 4 5 6
4	*Positive relations with others:*
	People would describe me as a giving person, willing to share my time with others
	1 2 3 4 5 6
5	*Purpose in life:*
	Some people wander aimlessly through life, but I am not one of them
	1 2 3 4 5 6
6	*Self-acceptance:*
	I like most aspects of my personality
	1 2 3 4 5 6

Table 6.2 Example statements from each of the six areas of the Ryff Scale (reproduced by kind permission of Carol Ryff)

others, while a low score suggests the individual has few close, trusting relationships with others.

Purpose in life

A high score in purpose in life reveals the individual has goals in life and a sense of direction, while a low score suggests that the individual lacks a sense of meaning and a sense of direction in life.

Self-acceptance

A high score in self-acceptance indicates the individual has a positive attitude towards the self, while a low score suggests that the individual feels dissatisfied with self.

The Ryff PWBs must be used by someone who is conversant with the purpose of the tool, skilled in the interpretation of its scores and knowledgeable about how to use the data that it elicits.

Activity 6.1

Using the six areas of the Ryff Scale, identify a matching descriptor that depicts your personal psychological wellbeing.

Interventions to support and promote wellbeing

Over the years psychologists have devised and experimented with ways of helping people cope with psychological problems, as well as with ways of promoting psychological wellbeing interventions among individuals and groups. The success of the interventions has, however, been more commonly recorded for individuals than groups (Huppert and Bayliss, 2004). This is because, traditionally, psychologists work at an individual level, although work with groups is noticeably increasing. Either of two specific interventions can be used to support and promote wellbeing in individuals. The first is Mindfulness-based Cognitive Therapy (MBCT) and the second is Wellbeing Therapy (WBT).

Mindfulness-based cognitive therapy

Mindfulness, which has its origin in Eastern Buddhist meditation (Baer *et al.*, 2004), refers to an individual's awareness and intention to attend to personal ongoing experiences (Brown and Ryan, 2003; Kabat-Zinn, 2003). Brown and Ryan define mindfulness as the state of being attentive to and aware of what is taking place in the present. The use of mindfulness, in such present-moment awareness, can enhance affective balance and psychological wellbeing. It has been demonstrated to do so by preventing habitual reactions and encouraging a more adaptive and deliberate response to experiences (Baer *et al.*, 2004; Segal *et al.*, 2002). Mindfulness is a skill that can be learnt and developed through the meditation practice and can be increasingly beneficial for the practitioner. In particular, its practice at higher levels is found to be related to more positive affect (mood), life satisfaction, self-esteem and optimism and to less negative affect and rumination (going over negative thoughts again and again) (Brown and Ryan, 2003). It is also useful in the reduction of stress, especially when it is used in combination with exercises, sitting and walking. Individuals are taught to recognise and attend to their distressing thoughts and emotions early, to disengage from thoughts that do not serve any purpose and to avoid behaviour patterns such as rumination and avoidance. Mindfulness-based interventions are effective in improving the psychological wellbeing in individuals with a wide range of conditions. They can, for example, relieve anxiety, depression and panic attacks. Brown and Ryan found that individuals who had greater ability to be mindful had a significant decrease in mood disturbance and equally a significant improvement in their wellbeing.

Wellbeing therapy

Wellbeing therapy is an intervention specifically aimed at enhancing psychological wellbeing (Ruini and Fava, 2009). It takes the technique of Cognitive Behaviour Therapy (CBT) as its base and builds on it using Ryff's (1989) six dimensions of psychological wellbeing. The obvious success in the reduction of some psychological problems such as anxiety and depression has been acknowledged through the technique of CBT. Although CBT is now an established approach – it is used on its own or in combination with drug treatment – for the relief of some psychological distress and psychological disorders such as anxiety and depression, WBT is claimed to be an improved approach. It has an added advantage over CBT in that it is a relatively short-term intervention for the restoration, improvement and maintenance of wellbeing, including the management of anxiety and depression. CBT is commonly delivered over a period of months and deals only with psychological conditions.

WBT emphasises self-observation with the use of a structured diary and is directive and people-oriented. It uses an educational model in that it aims to induce learning in the individual as it is progressively delivered. It is designed to extend over eight sessions, which may take place every week or every other week. The duration of each session may range from 30 to 50 minutes. The eight sessions are roughly divided into three stages – initial, intermediate and final – and each stage is made up of two or three sessions. The initial sessions are aimed at helping the individual identify episodes of wellbeing in their life and setting these episodes in a situational context, no matter how short-lived they were. The intermediate sessions encourage the individual to identify thoughts and beliefs that led to premature interruption of wellbeing. During the final sessions, Ryff's six dimensions are progressively introduced to the individual as long as the material which is recorded lends itself to them. For example, the therapist may be in a position to explain that autonomy comprises independence and self-determination, or that personal growth comprises being open to new experience and considering self as expanding over time.

The intervention aims to change attitudes and beliefs that are detrimental to wellbeing, to stimulate personal growth and to reinforce wellbeing. It also encourages self-help and exposure. The goal for the health practitioner is to lead the individual from an impaired level to an optimal level in the six dimensions of psychological wellbeing.

CONCLUSION

There is a strong relationship between the concepts of health and wellbeing, as both concepts basically consider the same psychological, sociological and physical components of human experience. However, health has its focus on the physical aspect of this experience in the main, while wellbeing places an emphasis on psychological issues that influence an individual's overall state of being, which ultimately includes physical health. Consequently, it is the state of psychological wellbeing that must be logically assessed by health practitioners using such established instruments as Ryff's long scale. The data derived from such instruments can be used in the two specific interventions, MBCT and WBT, which are found to be beneficial for both the restoration and promotion of psychological wellbeing.

Further reading

Feldman, F. (2004) *Pleasure and the Good Life*. Gloucestershire: Clarendon Press

This book provides a very good introduction to the hedonistic life. It critiques the impact on individuals' wellbeing and questions how individuals assess 'the good life'.

Kiefer, R.A. (2008) 'An integrative review of the concept of wellbeing'. *Holistic Nursing Practice*, 22 (05): 242–52

This paper discusses the health-related behaviour dimensions which are relevant to the facets that make up wellbeing.

Kraut, R. (2007) *What is Good and Why*. Cambridge, MA: Harvard University Press

This book presents a lucid and wide-ranging discussion of the core ethical theories and provides an appealing set of answers to a range of ethical questions.

Raz, J. (2004) 'The role of wellbeing'. *Philosophical Perspectives*, 18: 269–94

This article discusses the role of wellbeing and the importance of objectivity, while providing an underpinning of how using subjective wellbeing can be utilised within concepts of wellbeing.

Ruini, C. and Fava, G.A. (2009) 'Wellbeing therapy for generalised anxiety disorder'. *Journal of Clinical Psychology*, 65 (05): 510–19

The authors discuss in some detail how wellbeing therapy is used in practice and how its effectiveness is evaluated.

Schickler, P. (2005) 'Achieving health or achieving wellbeing'. *Learning in Health and Social Care*, 4(4): 217–27

The author provides a substantial amount of up-to-date information on the similarities and differences between the concepts of health and wellbeing.

Chapter 7

Spirituality and Wellbeing

Anneyce Knight and Qaisra Khan

'To thine own self be true'
(William Shakespeare, *Hamlet* Act I, Scene 3, 78)

Learning outcomes

In this chapter you will learn how to:

- appreciate that there is diversity and uniqueness within the broad term of spirituality;

- explain the spectrum of spirituality;

- discuss religion, faith and belief in the UK, and in comparison with the Czech Republic;

- identify a range of tools for individuals and communities to access their spirituality and wellbeing.

INTRODUCTION

This chapter discusses spirituality and its relationship with wellbeing in the context of the UK, and also provides a short case study from the Czech Republic. Spirituality as a concept is explored and the notion of a spectrum of spirituality is discussed. Religion, faith and belief, as defined by the 2001 Census, are examined. The place of spirituality in health and social care service provision for enhancing wellbeing is considered, and the need for educating students and professionals in this area is debated. A range of tools for individuals and communities to access their spirituality and wellbeing is presented.

DEFINING SPIRITUALITY

The word 'spirituality' can lead to some confusion and bring about strong feelings. Its association with religion makes people either welcome or dismiss the term. For some the word is too fluffy and for others it provides the answers to life's questions. The word 'spirituality' is derived from the Latin for breath, *spiritus*. Breath is the vital or animating force within all living beings. The word 'spirituality' has gone on to mean so much more than just breath, evoking diverse reactions, although without doubt breathing is the essential foundation for maintaining life. While each person breathes and follows their individual life's journey, every human being is in certain aspects:

- 'Like all other people
- Like some other people
- Like no other person' (Swinton, 2001, p. 21).

Every person is like all other people because we are all human, coming into life gasping for air and with the certainty of death. It is the experience between birth and death that is so unique and makes each person unlike any other. Sharing an experience, such as loss, or similarities, such as gender, culture or religion, makes individuals like others who share those same connections.

It is this uniqueness of individuals that makes spirituality so difficult to define, yet it is both vital and animating as it is at every individual's core and gives them the power to define their lives and wellbeing. In *Spiritual Care Matters* (NHS Education for Scotland, 2009), the suggestion is made that instead of seeking a definitive definition of spirituality, each of us should relate to the human spirit within all of us; that human spirit and individuality that is searching for meaning, peace or hope. Individuals need the courage to accept themselves for who they are and that will give them the understanding to accept others for who they are. 'An expression of empathy, the sharing of family stories, hopes, fears, gestures, humour, sadness and an accepting recognition of culture, belief or faith' (NHS Education for Scotland, 2009, 14–15) can be conducive to wellbeing, as these factors are representative of the human spirit and, as such, they are spiritual. Thus, the acceptance of oneself and the acknowledgement and acceptance of others will give all the ability to live their lives being true to themselves, which will enhance their wellbeing in a profoundly spiritual way. Indeed, Ware (2009) states that while working with people at the end of their lives, people's most common regrets included, 'I wish I'd had the courage to live a life true to myself, not the life others expected of me' and 'I wish I'd had the courage to express my feelings'.

The first step to providing the space to learn to actively listen and recognise oneself and to accept oneself and others is to focus on breathing. Breathing is the stable solid ground that can provide a refuge regardless of individual thoughts and the world around (Plum Village, 2010). Moments focusing on breathing in and out will help everyone to discover what is important to them and how they connect to the world around them.

Activity 7.1

1. Pause and focus on breathing in and out:

- What are you aware of?
- What do you feel?

2. *The Values in Healthcare: a spiritual approach* (Janki Foundation for Global Health Care, 2004) has seven tools to help us to discover what our values are and what is important to us. One of the worksheets within the programme uses the following reflective tool and asks:

- Think of the songs you love. What values are reflected through the words and music?
- Think of poems, quotes, books that are important to you. What values are reflected in them?
- What images are important to you? Think of your favourite scenes, views, paintings or perhaps statues. What values and feelings do they evoke?

(Reproduced with kind permission of The Janki Foundation for Global Health Care.)

While doing these activities, remember that it is your response and values you are focusing on, and these are individual to you, so there is no right or wrong answer.

THE SPECTRUM OF SPIRITUALITY

Religion and spirituality have seemingly become synonymous. Religion, according to Koening *et al.* (2001, p. 18), 'is an organised system of beliefs, practices, rituals and symbols designed (a) to facilitate closeness to the sacred or transcendent (God, higher power, or ultimate truth/ reality) and (b) to foster an understanding of one's relationship and responsibility to others living in a community'. In contrast, they define spirituality as 'the personal quest for understanding answers to ultimate questions about life, about meaning, and about relationships to the sacred or transcendent, which may (or may not) lead to or arise from the development of religious rituals and the formation of community' (Koening *et al.*, 2001, p. 18).

In reality, however, there is a spectrum of spirituality, referred to not only by NHS Education for Scotland (2009) but also by others such as Dr Nigel Copsey who is responsible for spiritual, religious and cultural care in East London and the City Mental Health NHS Trust. At one end of the spectrum is 'religious experience', where someone may more readily be linked into a faith tradition, despite the diversity of their views within that tradition's beliefs and practices. At the other end of the spiritual spectrum are those who experience a deep sense and awareness of the spiritual dimension of life through the world around and within them. Dr Copsey further suggests that individuals may move along this spectrum in either direction throughout their lives. Therefore, it can be seen that religion and spirituality are distinct but not inseparable: part of the same scale, thereby meaning an individual's spirituality cannot be defined by just one word.

So at one end of the spiritual spectrum are those who use religious language and on the other those who talk of a sense of awe and wonder in response to nature, music or the arts that is beyond the immediate experience of life, and that gives to the person an inner sense of the mystery of life that transcends the rational (consider your responses to Activity 7.1). Many people have deeply transforming inner experiences. There are those who experience this type of inner journey in a deeply personal way, while others encounter the spiritual in the mystery of relationships with others. There are still others who look forward to a day when the 'old dogmas of religion no longer oppress rational thinkers' (NHS Education for Scotland, 2009, p. 6). Most people would probably inhabit the middle of the spectrum. These people may, according to Dr Copsey, be 'deeply spiritual in the orientation of their lives but would not align themselves to any faith group'. Having an appreciation of who and where we are on the spiritual spectrum is important to individual wellbeing (see also Chapter 3). As Dadi Janki, President of the Janki Foundation, said, 'It is only when you are standing on the foundation of your values that you are able to maintain your truth, no matter what the surrounding circumstances' (Janki Foundation for Global Health Care, 2010).

RELIGION, FAITH AND BELIEF IN THE UNITED KINGDOM

As has been shown, religion and spirituality are different, as an individual seeking spirituality wishes to understand their relationship to the world, and this may include developing a religious belief (Koenig *et al.*, 2001). However, religious belief or faith would still seem to have a place in contemporary society within the UK according to the 2001 Census which took place on 29 April that year. As part of this Census, the population was asked to voluntarily identify their religion with the question 'What is your religion?' (Office for National Statistics (ONS), 2003; Economic and Social Research Council (ESRC), 2010). This was the first time that this topic had been included in the Census for England, Wales and Scotland but it had been incorporated in censuses for Northern Ireland since 1861 (ONS, 2003; ESRC, 2010). It was a voluntary question because there had been concerns raised by the UK Parliament relating to civil liberties (ESRC, 2010). There was a 92 per cent response rate, which suggests that the majority of the population were happy to answer the question and did not see it as an infringement of their civil liberties (ONS, 2003). As the question only identifies a person's affiliation to a specific denomination, it does not identify the level of an individual's religiousness or spirituality. Thus, there will be individual differences between those who affiliate themselves with a specific denomination. Nevertheless, the Census data do provide an indication that 92 per cent of the UK population recognise that they are on the spiritual spectrum.

Table 7.1 shows the percentage of the population who declared a religious faith in the 2001 Census.

Within the 2001 Census, there seemed to be a geographical correlation between people identifying themselves with a religion both nationally and regionally. In Northern Ireland 86 per cent of the population identified their religion, which was 9 per cent higher than in England and Wales, and 19 per cent higher than in Scotland (ONS, 2003). However, this higher identification with a religion may have been due to the fact that the population of Northern Ireland has historically always

Religion	Per cent
Christian	71.6
Muslim	2.7
Hindu	1.0
Sikh	0.6
Jewish	0.5
Buddhist	0.3
Other religions	0.3
No religion stated	23.2

Table 7.1 Religious make-up of the UK population, 2001 (Source: ONS, 2003)

been asked about their religious beliefs in the Census. The populations of Scotland and Northern Ireland were additionally asked to identify the religion of their upbringing.

Also of note is that of the 23.2 per cent who did not state a religion, 16 per cent defined themselves using such terms as agnostic, atheists and heathens, thereby indicating that they have self-awareness as they know who they are, their values and their connection with the world (ONS, 2003). 0.75 per cent of the 23.2 per cent identified themselves as 'Jedi Knight', an answer promoted by a contemporaneous internet campaign to have Jedi recognised as an official religion (ONS, 2003). It will be interesting to compare the data presented in this section with the data from the 2011 Census as there are no comparative data from the 1991 Census.

Case study 7.1 Spirituality and religion in the Czech Republic

The degree of religiosity was small and rapidly decreasing in the Czech Republic during the time of the communist regime, even in comparison with other Eastern Bloc countries. On the other hand, in the late 1980s, a part of society had high expectations for Christianity (mainly the Catholic Church), which were supposed to be met after the fall of the regime that occurred during the Velvet Revolution in 1989. The canonisation of St Agnes of Bohemia in 1989 and the subsequent visit of the Pope to Czechoslovakia was seen as a manifestation of the power of Czech Christianity and, at the same time, a demonstration of protest against the anti-religious regime. Indeed, the beginning of the 1990s was actually committed to the revival of faith in the Czech Republic. The only religious organisations that were not affected by the decline in religiosity were small Christian churches and sects but they counted as barely 0.5 per cent of the total population.

The weakening influence of traditional religion does not mean that the Czechs are becoming less religious; it means that another type of spirituality is influential. The Czech people do not reject the supernatural as a whole, but rather traditional religious systems and organised religion in general. This would seem to support the argument that there is a spectrum of spirituality. It seems that private and individual approaches are much more important than church-organised forms of piety: for example, private prayer at home or accessing more mystical forms of spirituality such as tarot cards. Given that the Czech Republic is considered to be one of the most secularised countries, this is not surprising. In fact, there was a similar situation more than 100 years ago and that is why it is not assumed that the current situation is a consequence of the 40 years of the communist regime.

However, a large number of people do consider themselves to be Catholics or Protestants and members of churches and some attend religious services. Also, according to the 2001 Census, 50 per cent of the Czech population believe in amulets and horoscopes and 70 per cent believe in predictions of the future. Given that these types of privatised 'mystical' religions are in favour with the younger generation and the more educated within the population, this trend will probably increase and illustrates the spectrum of spirituality in Czechoslovakia.

Private forms of spirituality influence not only religious life but also economic life. Christian missions have gradually developed a promotional campaign in order to obtain other 'consumers', and the Christian life began to manifest itself as a parliamentary lobby and was used in an effort to obtain funding from various governmental and non-governmental organisations. The whole business community in the Czech Republic has begun to focus on fulfilling the spiritual needs of individuals. This suggests that there is an acceptance that spirituality is more than religion and has a place throughout Czech society.

With thanks to Dr Marie Mackova, University of Masaryk, Brno, Czech Republic.
Source: Nešpor.Z.R. a kol.(2008) Příručka sociologie náboženství. Praha: Slon

THE PLACE OF SPIRITUALITY IN HEALTH AND SOCIAL CARE SERVICE PROVISION

Reference has been made to the link between spirituality and health in research, but this has more often been seen in relation to the connection between religion and health (Koenig *et al.*, 2001). For example, Ridge *et al.* (2008) state that religion is a supportive strategy for many African people who face major adverse life events such as challenges to wellness, immigration issues and poverty. Nevertheless, research has also shown that assessing the patient's/client's spirituality and providing appropriate support can provide positive outcomes for patients/clients (Koenig *et al.*, 2001). Indeed, the wider concept of spirituality is seen as important within the UK health system in, for example, the areas of mental health, cancer and palliative care. In mental health practice it has been recognised that 'spirituality can help people maintain good mental health. It can help them cope with everyday stress and can keep them grounded. Tolerant and inclusive spiritual communities can provide valuable support and friendship' (Mental Health Foundation, 2007, p. 4). Faith and spirituality can therefore be seen to be a key factor in enhancing mental health while maintaining individual mental wellbeing and promoting social inclusion for those who are marginalised from economic, social and cultural activities (NHS Education for Scotland, 2009; European Commission, 2004).

Within cancer and palliative care service provision, the National Institute for Health and Clinical Excellence (NICE) made a key recommendation for the availability of sensitive spiritual support services to be provided by staff who are responsive to both patients' and carers' spiritual needs, as part of their guidance in *Improving Supportive and Palliative Care for Adults: The Manual* (NICE, 2004). NICE identifies that the support provided can range from 'an informal sharing of ideas about the ultimate purpose of existence to the provision of a formalised religious ritual' (NICE, 2004, p. 96). For example, one person with cancer stated that for her 'the most useful support was The Haven in Fulham; I like the idea of people to contact although it wasn't me who talked about it [spirituality]'.

From these examples, it can be seen that spirituality has a place as part of the holistic care provided by all health and social care professionals. Indeed, spiritual care is the essence of the work of these professionals and, according to NHS Education for Scotland (2009, p. 4), 'it enables and promotes healing in the fullest sense to all parties, both giver and receiver, of such care'. From this, the importance of knowing oneself can be seen in order to achieve a positive outcome and a sense of wellbeing for all. To attain this, health and social care professionals need to be educated appropriately. Training by spiritual care staff and chaplaincy does occur for practitioners, but this has been seen as limited in terms of its effect and recommendations have been made for specialist culturally competent staff to meet patients'/clients' individual spiritual and religious needs (NHS Education for Scotland, 2009). However, this approach would seem to limit the availability of spiritual support, so ongoing education should be provided to all in health and social care, both to undergraduates and practitioners, in order to maximise spiritual wellbeing, not only for themselves but also for their patients and clients. Culliford (2009) provides a model for teaching spiritual values and skills to third-year medical students, a model that he sees as transferable to other health care (and social care) professionals. He emphasises the importance of revitalising the bond between medicine, healing and spirituality through education to promote patient/client wellbeing.

TOOLS FOR INDIVIDUALS AND COMMUNITIES TO ACCESS THEIR SPIRITUALITY AND WELLBEING

There is a variety of tools available for individuals and communities to access their spirituality and wellbeing, apart from directly accessing faith communities and their holy books. Some are discussed in this section.

Mindfulness, prayer and meditation

As mentioned above, a key tool to accessing spirituality and wellbeing is to breathe. Whatever term is used, mindfulness, prayer and meditation all give individuals the precious time to stop whatever they are doing and just be still and live in the moment. For example, as the Plum Village website states:

> We do not need to control our breath. Feel the breath as it actually is. It may be long or short, deep or shallow. With our awareness it will naturally become slower and deeper. Conscious breathing is the key to uniting body and mind and bringing the energy of mindfulness into each moment of our life. We may like to recite:
> Breathing in I know that I am breathing in.
> Breathing out I know that I am breathing out. (Plum Village, 2010)

The Plum Village Meditation Practice Centre was founded by Thich Nhat Hanh (Thây), a Vietnamese Buddhist monk who founded the Unified Buddhist Church in 1969. It provides a place for a retreat and resources that will help people on the path to mindfulness. Some useful resources include books written by Thây, for example *The Energy of Prayer: how to deepen your spiritual practice*, *Taming the Tiger Within*, *Meditations on Transforming Difficult Emotions* and *The Blooming of a Lotus: guided meditation for achieving the miracle of mindfulness*. Other traditions also emphasise reflection, meditation and prayer, such as monasticism and asceticism in Christianity and Hinduism.

The exploration of spirituality by some traditions

The Janki Foundation for Global Health Care has a number of tools for individuals to reflect and discover what their values are and what is most important to them. As well as *Values in Healthcare: a spiritual approach*, mentioned in Activity 7.1, the organisation, together with the British Holistic Medical Association, has published *The Heart of Wellbeing: seven tools for surviving and thriving* by Jan Alcoe and edited by Craig Brown. This book and CD explores the need for individuals to deal with the physical, mental, emotional and spiritual aspects of their lives to enhance their wellbeing.

The Threshold Society (**www.sufism.org**) is a non-profit educational foundation. The society is affiliated with the Mevlevi Order, and offers training programmes, seminars and retreats around the world. These are intended to provide a structure for practice and study within Sufism. Sufism is the application of spiritual principles to achieve full spiritual development for oneself in synergy with one's community. Some useful resources written by Kabir Helminsky include *Living Presence: a Sufi way to mindfulness and the essential self*.

Five-a-day for positive mental health and wellbeing

The five-a-day for positive mental health and wellbeing is a useful holistic tool, particularly since spiritual and physical health and wellbeing are linked. Foresight, the Government's Office for Science, was tasked to explore ways to take advantage of and increase the mental capital and wellbeing in the UK in order to benefit both individuals and society as a whole. Foresight identified that for positive mental health, spirituality was a key part, alongside the emotional, psychological, social and physical factors (Foresight, 2008). Evidence presented to this Foresight project by the NEF Centre for Wellbeing identified 'Five Ways to Wellbeing'. These are:

- Connect ... with the people around you. With family, friends, colleagues and neighbours. At home, work or school in your local community. Think of these as cornerstones of your life and invest time in developing them. Building these connections will support and enrich you every day.

- Be active ... go for a walk or a run. Step outside. Cycle. Play a game. Garden. Dance. Exercising makes you feel good. Most importantly, discover a physical activity you enjoy and that suits your level of mobility and fitness.
- Take notice ... be curious. Catch sight of something beautiful. Remark on the unusual. Notice the changing seasons. Savour the moment, whether you are walking to work, eating lunch or talking to friends. Be aware of the world around you and what you are feeling. Reflecting on your experiences will help you appreciate what matters to you.
- Learn ... try something new. Rediscover old interests. Sign up for a course. Take on a different responsibility at work. Fix a bike. Learn to play an instrument or how to cook your favourite food. Set a challenge that you enjoy achieving. Learning new things will make you more confident as well as being fun.
- Give ... do something nice for a friend or a stranger. Thank someone. Smile. Volunteer your time. Join a community group. Look out, as well as in. Seeing yourself, and your happiness, as linked to the wider community can be incredibly rewarding and creates connections with the people around you. (Aked *et al.*, 2008, p. 1)

These five ways to wellbeing all increase self-awareness and are, in effect, spiritual activities. Whatever an individual's belief, it is useful to ask how these actions help them to develop their spirituality and wellbeing.

Case study 7.2 Martial arts, spirituality and wellbeing

I have studied martial arts for 25 years. Martial arts training means being active and going through a whole range of movements and exercises. All parts of the mind and body are used in an ever-increasing level of fitness, creating an understanding of how one's body works and enhancing mind/body connectivity in the pursuit of excellence. This includes fitness of the body, flexibility, inner calmness of spirit, an uncluttered mind and overall wellbeing of both mind and body. Martial arts cultivate a mind which is forever learning and yet performs moving Zen meditation which empties the mind. When the mind is empty it can think properly, is uncluttered and gives the individual a calmness of spirit. After every martial arts session you feel cleansed and your mind and body are refreshed, recharged and at peace with the world. It is said that a martial artist in full flow can sense everything around him and empties his mind to take in all noise, movements and to react naturally without thinking about any action. To me martial arts allow one to connect with nature and the natural world and people and increase my spiritual wellbeing. (Allan Prasad, Sensei)

The media

The BBC has a large quantity of web resources and programming that relates to spirituality, which can be accessed through various sites including **www.bbc.co.uk/religion** This includes information on a diverse range of faith traditions and a message board covering a variety of topics. In addition, the BBC offers an array of programmes such as the six-part series presented by Mark Easton in 2006 that explored themes to understand what lasting happiness is. There are also radio programmes, such as *Something Understood*, covering ethical and religious discussion that takes a spiritual theme and explores it through music, prose and poetry.

Literature

Books

It can be useful to read books on spirituality, particularly those written by spiritual practitioners and by those who have been on a journey. For example, *The Spiral Staircase*, a memoir by Karen Armstrong. This is a spellbinding autobiography in which Karen relates her journey from a Roman Catholic convent to when she began her writing career and her focus on the sacred texts of Judaism, Christianity and Islam. Reading the personal story of how someone else has lived with despair, discouragement and disappointment can provide one with a sense of connectedness and inspiration. Other titles include:

- *Bilal* by Hal Craig. An inspiring book in which the author gives Bilal a voice to tell his own story. Now an old man in Damascus, he had been an Ethiopian slave who went on to become the first muezzin in Islam, and was therefore the first person to recite the words that are now repeated daily in mosques around the world.
- *The Five People you Meet in Heaven* by Mitch Albom. This is an interesting reflection on life and death and the people we meet in it. The first person that is met in heaven is someone the main character does not know but on whose life they had a major impact.

- *The Celestine Prophecy: an adventure* by James Redfield. At one level it is an adventure story and on another level it is about the lessons learnt along the way.

Prayer books, poems or spiritual texts

- *The Prophet* by Kahil Gibran is a series of philosophical poetic essays which discuss a selection of life issues.
- *Transcendence Prayer of People of Faith* edited by Daniel Faivre and Tony McCaffry. This text contains prayers and poems from a variety of traditions on the subject of the divine.
- *Seasons of Life: prose and poetry for secular ceremonies and private reflection,* compiled by Nigel Collins, is helpful from a secular perspective.

CONCLUSION

This chapter has demonstrated that no discussion on spirituality can exclude religion as these two subjects are interwoven and both continue to have a place both in the UK and the Czech Republic. A spectrum of spirituality has been identified, along which individuals travel in either direction during their lifetime, and for each individual this is a unique and individual experience. Without a doubt, individuals need to know themselves in order to maximise their own wellbeing and in order that they can maximise the wellbeing of others. In order to achieve this we all need to be open to other people. Furthermore, it has been identified that assessing spirituality is an essential component of wellbeing and a method is needed to assess individual wellbeing within health and social care service provision. One barrier to promoting spiritual wellbeing is a lack of self-awareness by health and social care professionals, which education should seek to address. A variety of tools is available for individuals, health and social care professionals and communities to explore their spirituality and no one approach holds higher merit than another.

With grateful thanks to Dr Nigel Copsey of East London and the City Mental Health NHS Trust and to Allan Prasad.

Further reading and websites

Koenig, H.G., McCullough, M.E. and Larson, D.B. (2001) *Handbook of Religion and Health*. Oxford: Oxford University Press

A useful text discussing spirituality and religion, and linking religion to a wide range of wellbeing and health issues, although it has a USA focus.

Inter Faith Network for the UK **www.interfaith.org.uk**

This organisation was set up to promote 'good relations between people of different faiths' and the website includes details of some useful publications.

Part 3: Physical Aspects of Wellbeing

Chapter 8

Food and Wellbeing

Stuart Spear

Learning outcomes

In this chapter you will learn how to:

- understand the role of food in individual health and wellbeing;

- develop an awareness of the impact of food production on ecological public health;

- identify the impact of private food businesses on public policy in respect of health and wellbeing.

This chapter looks at the relationship between food and wellbeing. It considers the ways in which new scientific evidence reveals a link between food and mental wellbeing by looking at some of the research that appeared in June and July 2010. It notes that little of this evidence is applied at a policy level, while public health campaign groups argue that growing mental ill health is linked to our modern diet. The chapter then looks at how physical wellbeing is threatened by rising obesity rates. It investigates some government policies over the past ten years to tackle obesity both locally and nationally. The chapter also looks at wellbeing through the prism of ecological public health, citing an example of how human and planetary wellbeing are connected through our relationship with food.

INTRODUCTION

Over recent months (2011) wellbeing has risen up the political agenda. 'The Big Society', David Cameron's announcement of a wellbeing index (Stratton, 2010), the planned establishment of Health and Wellbeing

Boards under NHS reforms (Department of Health, 2010), and the government's realisation that it can no longer afford the levels of mental ill health prevalent in the UK (HM Government, 2010) have all raised the profile of wellbeing.

The Department of Health recognises that population-based wellbeing can be improved through, among other things, housing, our built environment and workplace stress. Unfortunately, despite the growing evidence that food is integral to our wellbeing, both through its impact on mental health and physical health, it appears to be slipping off the political agenda. Here we explore how the link between mental ill health and food is failing to figure at policy level while, despite a plethora of initiatives over the last decade, obesity still remains a major killer.

WHAT WE EAT AND OUR MENTAL HEALTH

'We are what we eat', goes the old adage, and the brain, being the largest organ in our body, is as much affected by our diet as our heart or liver. The problem with the brain as compared with the heart is its complexity. We know there is a link between a diet too rich in fats or salt and cardiovascular disease, we understand the link between liver damage and alcohol. But making that link between our mental health and what we eat is proving a much tougher challenge.

The evidence of a link

There is no shortage of research. Evidence appears from around the world almost weekly supporting the link between what we eat and mental health. For example, in July 2010, researchers in Pittsburgh found a link between high-fat diets and changes in dopamine, a chemical in the brain that controls our reward system (Society for the Study of Ingestive Behaviour, 2010). The findings suggest that diet affects the neurochemistry in the brain that regulates motivation.

Another study in the same month from Australia found a possible link between Attention Deficit Hyperactivity Disorder (ADHD) in adolescents and Western diets (Halliday, 2010). Researchers from Perth's Telethon Institute for Child Health Research studied 1800 adolescents, categorising their diets as 'healthy' – high in fresh fruit, vegetables and oily fish – and 'Western' – tending towards takeaway food, confectionery and processed foods. The researchers found that those eating the 'Western' diet ran more than double the risk of suffering ADHD when compared with those with a 'healthy' diet.

Researchers at the University of Montreal published results in the *Journal of Clinical Psychiatry* from the largest clinical study ever conducted on treating depression with Omega 3. The study found that Omega 3 improved the symptoms for those suffering depression but not those with an anxiety disorder (Lesperance *et al.*, 2010).

US researchers concluded in an article in the *Journal of Policy Analysis and Management* that schoolchildren participating in the National School Lunch Programme were gaining a significant increase in educational opportunity and attainments (Carland-Adams, 2010). In Stockholm, Sweden, a study published in the *Journal of Alzheimer's Disease* found that the presence of higher levels of all the vitamin E forms provides a reduced risk of developing Alzheimer's (Manglalasche *et al.*, 2010). These examples are just the tip of the iceberg. It is almost as though we are being sandblasted with evidence, and yet persuading policy makers of the link between diet and mental health is proving a tough task.

The UK situation

In a study on the link between food and behaviour published by the Mental Health Foundation and Sustain (the alliance for better food and farming), an attempt has been made to address whether a substantial increase in mental ill health is linked to changes in human diet (Van de Weyer, 2005). Currently in the UK, one in six adults at any one time suffer some form of mental ill health, while one in four of us will have a mental health problem at some point in our lives (HM Government, 2010). The Department of Health has over the last two years been investigating what lies behind these figures and has, under New Labour's *New Horizons* strategy and now the coalition government's public mental health strategy, been trying to reduce the £22.5 billion it costs the NHS each year to treat mental ill health. When you factor in lost days in sickness, the economic cost rockets to £77 billion a year (HM Government, 2010). The WHO calculates that mental disorder is responsible for 22.8 per cent of the disease burden in the UK, compared with 15.9 per cent for cancer and 16.2 per cent for cardiovascular disease (WHO, 2008). *New Horizons* lists poor housing, workplace stress, alcohol and drug misuse, climate change, lack of green spaces and our built environment as potential causes of mental ill health. Food gets one mention and then only in terms of breastfeeding and nutrition (HM Government, 2010).

However, Sustain and the Mental Health Foundation tell a different story. Our diet has evolved through history. The agricultural revolution, the industrial revolution, world trade, world wars and the time constraints imposed by modernity have all impacted on what we eat. Ironically it is during the rationing of the Second World War that most nutritionists agree we were at our healthiest. Rationing provided low-income families with sufficient protein and vitamins while, no matter who you were, meats, fats and sugars were in short supply.

Since 1942 the Government has been collecting data on what we eat. We learn from these that since the nutritionally halcyon days of the 1940s we are now consuming vastly more meat and processed food, while eating about 34 per cent fewer vegetables, with fish consumption down by about 59 per cent. Consumption of saturated fats, salts and refined sugar has risen, while our intake of Vitamin A, riboflavin, iodine, magnesium and potassium have all dropped below recommended levels (Van de Weyer, 2005). Factor in our increased consumption of processed foods, trans fats, food production chemicals, artificial sweeteners, pesticides and antibiotics and you create a heady stew of chemicals, all reacting with each other and all affecting us in a way which is impossible to calculate.

When you combine this with the almost weekly evidence emerging that what we eat impacts mental health, and the evidence documented in the Sustain report (Van de Weyer, 2005) confirming that link, then the report's conclusion that what we eat may contribute to rising mental ill health makes uncomfortable reading.

Conclusion from Van de Weyer (2005) *Changing Diets Changing Minds: how food affects mental wellbeing and behaviour.*

The result of these changes has been a rise in serious health problems that are in part attributed to the modern diet, including obesity, coronary heart disease, diabetes, cancer, osteoporosis and dental caries. Other problems, such as rising levels of some cancers, may be linked to some chemicals added to our food but a causal link is very difficult to establish.

Coupling this with the evidence presented in previous chapters raises the obvious question. Is it possible that the same changes that are contributing to our rising physical health problems are also contributing to our rising mental health problems? (p. 84)

WHAT WE EAT AND OUR PHYSICAL HEALTH

Clearly food plays a key role in our health and therefore our wellbeing. It was the Boer War that first revealed the scale of ill health in Britain. Between 1899 and 1902, faced with potential defeat by Boer farmers, recruiting sergeants were rejecting about 60 per cent of volunteers on the grounds of rickets, stunted growth, poor eyesight, deformities and weight. Subsequent inquiries into the nation's 'physical deterioration' sparked a hot debate: what role should the state play in influencing what people eat? It is a debate that rages today, with ministers of all parties fearful of being accused of 'nanny statism' when pushing for better nutrition, while food companies argue foods high in sugar and fats should be available to allow people indulgences in what may otherwise be healthy diets. Thus, it was around the early part of this century that our relationship with food shifted significantly. Tobacco companies had up to this point been the number one enemy of public health, then worrying new figures began to emerge.

The obesity threat

By 2000, most adults in England were overweight, while one in five, eight million in total, were obese. Obesity rates had trebled by 1980, with obesity killing 30 000 a year and shortening lives on average by nine years (Committee of Public Accounts, 2002). But it was statistics relating to children that really focused minds. The annual health survey for 2004 revealed that one in four 11 to 15 year-olds was now obese, and that obesity prevalence for the period 1995 to 2004 had increased from 14 per cent to 24 per cent for boys and 15 per cent to 26 per cent for girls (NHS Information Centre, 2006). The obesity time bomb described by Chief Medical Officer Liam Donaldson in his 2002 CMO report was ticking (DH Chief Medical Officer, 2002). In the same year the House of Commons Health Committee reported obesity was about to knock tobacco off as the biggest killer in this country (House of Commons, 2004). A shift in government policy was needed to address this new threat.

The national response to obesity

The two government agencies tasked with delivering change were the Food Standards Agency (FSA) set up in 2000 in the wake of the BSE (commonly known as mad-cow disease) crisis, and the Department of Health (DH). Food safety up to this point had focused on *E. coli*, campylobacter, listeria and salmonella as the killers to combat. Fats, sugars and salts were now claiming far more lives than pathogens. In 2005, the FSA included the following goal as one of its key aims in its five-year strategic plan: 'to make it easier for all consumers to choose a healthy diet and thereby improve quality of life by reducing diet-related disease' (FSA, 2004).

The FSA then took a strategic decision. Rather than recommend that the government should force food companies to cut salts and fats, the agency chose to work with and influence food manufacturers by looking at ways of reformulating foods, while at the same time raising public awareness and so increasing demand for healthier foods. A key part of its strategy was the introduction of a clear nutrition signposting system that informs consumers about exactly what they are eating. It recommended the traffic light system as the most easily understood by consumers, alerting them to foods high in salt, fat and sugar with a red light on the packaging. While some retailers such as Asda, Sainsbury's and Waitrose introduced versions of the traffic light system, two of the largest retailers, Tesco and Morrisons, were adamantly opposed to the scheme, arguing that red would mean 'don't buy'. Instead, guidelines for daily amounts were introduced which, FSA research argued, consumers found confusing. It was the start of a dispute that would cause friction between business and the FSA and would ultimately lead to the FSA being stripped of its nutrition role in October 2010 (Lawrence, 2010).

With 75 per cent of the salt we eat already in the foods we buy, voluntary salt targets were set in 2006, most of which have been met by the major food manufacturers. New targets have now been set in an attempt to get average salt consumption down to 6 grammes a day (FSA, 2010). Reformulation did not just look at cutting salt and fat content, but used food science to produce healthier food without altering taste.

Meanwhile, the government was committed to halting the year-on-year rise in obesity in children under 11 by 2010 (House of Commons, 2006). The DH started working nationally and locally to promote healthy eating among the young while promoting healthy diets in local communities, workplaces and the NHS. At a national level the Five-a-Day campaign was now taking off and by 2006 the DH was licensing hundreds of products to carry the Five-a-Day logo.

The local response

However, despite these initiatives, there was a glaring hole in the strategy. No one was talking to the tens of thousands of independent high street Chinese takeaways, kebab shops, curry houses and fish and chip shops that provide a large proportion of the two billion takeaway meals we eat each year (Spear, 2008). Yet, evidence was starting to emerge that some of these foods were the worst culprits. One of the first pieces of research to emerge around the nutritional content of our high street takeaways was from Liverpool. Greater Merseyside has some of the highest rates of coronary disease in the country, killing 30 per cent more men and 20 per cent more women than the national average (Heart of Mersey, 2005). The statistics prompted the council's trading standards department to look at the nutritional value of foods served by the thousands of sole traders that had until now slipped under the public health radar. What they found was shocking. Fish and chips, pizzas, kebabs and, in particular, Chinese takeaway contained on average two days' salt content and, in one case, almost five times the recommended daily salt intake in one meal (Spear, 2008). Unlike in supermarkets, there was no way for a consumer to make healthy choices. The same meal in different outlets could contain vastly different levels of salt, sugar and fat.

There was no reason to believe that the Liverpool findings were any different elsewhere and so dozens of local authority initiatives began to spring up around the country to tackle these high-risk foods. These initiatives became known as the 'take away movement' (Spear, 2010). What makes this movement unique is that rather than just trying to persuade people to eat healthier foods, it takes the foods people want to eat and makes them healthier. In Wigan, for example, the council worked with the local primary care trust (PCT) to look at how deep frying could be made healthier. The type of oil you use, the temperature you fry at, the frequency of times you change the oil, whether the chip tray has holes, and even the frequency that you shake the frying food, all impact on the amount of fat finally left on the foods. Even the way that potatoes are stored can affect how much oil they absorb. The FSA later developed some of this work by producing advice sheets for caterers nationally on healthier frying techniques (FSA, 2010).

Other examples include a community garden project that was set up in Daventry, and a number of other councils encouraged allotment usage. In Gateshead the council cut salt consumption by 60 per cent by distributing salt shakers with five rather than 17 holes (Food Vision, 2009).

Case study 8.1 Gateshead salt shaker study

Gateshead Council's food control team noticed excessive salt being added to takeaway foods. So, in line with the FSA priority on reducing salt intake, the aim was to try to reduce salt usage at the point of sale.

The aim

To tie in with the FSA national reduced salt intake campaign and so improve health.

Objectives

- To determine the amount of salt added to food at hot food takeaways, at the point of sale (fish and chip shops chosen as a representative part of the sector).
- To determine the type of salt pot that is in general use at these premises.
- To confirm the amount of salt that is dispensed by salt pots of this type.
- To carry out experiments to determine how the problem of excessive salt being dispensed can be overcome by design.
- To design a new salt pot cap that dispenses significantly less salt.
- To work with the main supplier of the salt pots to fund the manufacture and supply of 1000 new-style caps and original salt pot bodies.
- To visit targeted businesses to give them free new-style caps and original salt pot bodies.
- To raise awareness about the project and health messages with targeted businesses and the public.
- To promote the availability of the new salt pot caps with the main local supplier.

Partners

- Some of the businesses in Gateshead that would help to focus on the main issues, business needs and possible improvement options.
- The public analyst to advise on sampling and carry out analysis for added salt.

- A major local supplier of equipment, materials and sundries to the catering trade.
- Collaboration with the main national supplier of the most commonly used salt pots by hot food takeaway businesses to work on the design and manufacture of 1000 new caps (and original salt pot bodies).
- Gateshead Council cabinet members who supported the aims of the project.

Methodology

Samples taken from 13 fish and chip shops across Gateshead were submitted to the public analyst, who reported between 1.34 g/portion to 3.90 g/portion. It was found that by filling holes and leaving a single ring of only five holes, the amount of salt dispensed was reduced by over 60 per cent.

The council worked with the main national supplier to get 1000 five-hole caps made. Fifty-two fish and chip shops were then consulted. Each business was visited and given leaflets, a poster and free salt pots with new caps. The cost savings of using less salt were explained. The response was very positive. The cost of food sampling analysis and of manufacturing the 1000 new tops was met from the food sampling budget with a contribution from the partner company.

Evaluation

Twenty per cent of businesses were contacted. All continued using the new pots and are satisfied with the amount of salt dispensed from the pots. They are all using much less salt. They accept that the original 17-hole caps dispersed too much salt and see the benefit of using less salt and having less waste.

Lessons learnt

There were no real obstacles or problems to be overcome. Businesses were pleased that we [Gateshead Council] were providing something 'free of charge' for use. Only five out of 52 visited showed some scepticism but then agreed to try the new salt pot design.

Public sector spending cuts

Then, with nutrition initiatives in place at a national and local level, the public sector spending cuts hit (2010). The fear is that many local authorities will now only be able to afford to perform statutory duties and so will shelve much of their nutrition work. This, combined with the England FSA handing responsibility for nutrition to the DH on 1 October 2010, means public health campaigners are waiting to see what will happen next in the battle to cut obesity rates.

All the signs are that health minister Andrew Lansley plans to place business at the heart of the obesity strategy. As one of the five 'responsibility deals' set up to tackle food, alcohol, physical activity, health at work and behaviour change, Lansley is inviting major food manufacturers to help shape policy on obesity (Lawrence, 2010). Public health campaigners fear that shareholder commitments will prove a major obstacle to introducing the kind of changes needed to drive down rising obesity rates.

We will have to wait and see whether returning to the pre-FSA days, when business played a greater role in government policy, will prove any more effective than the last ten-year strategy of persuading business to change. The same question is as relevant today as it was a hundred years ago: what role should the state play in influencing what people eat?

Activity 8.1 Wellbeing and physical health

There is currently a move by government to place business at the heart of policy making on nutrition.

- Can business meet the demands of its shareholders while also recommending policies for the public good?
- What benefits do you think business can bring to the obesity agenda?

FOOD WELLBEING AND THE ENVIRONMENT

In this section we will look at the relationship between food and wellbeing through the prism of the emerging paradigm of ecological public health (see the definition below). This approach sees human and planetary health as linked, with food acting as one of the most important connectors. Rethinking our relationship to the environment and applying ecological principles to the way we live and work has the potential to improve overall community health (McCallum, 2005). The argument goes that the more aware we become of the impact our actions have on the environment the more we understand our relationship with the world around us, including our communities. As we connect with our communities so we develop social capital, which in turn leads to wellbeing.

A definition of ecological public health (Nurse *et al.*, 2010)

Ecological public health is the science, art and politics of promoting human and environmental health and wellbeing, by enhancing:

- **Networks** – interconnections and common solutions;
- **Partnerships** – environmental and wider determinants;
- **Cycles** – life course and system approaches;
- **Balance** – health, environmental and inequalities impact assessments.

One recent example of how the environment, wellbeing and community can come together over food exists in the Belgian city of Ghent where, in May 2009, its 200 000 population chose to go voluntarily meat-and-fish-free every Thursday. Ghent claims to be the first city in Europe to try to go entirely vegetarian for a day a week in the fight against obesity and global warming (Traynor, 2009).

For the UK government, the relationship between meat consumption and climate change is a thorny issue that provides a conflict of interest. A four-year investigation by the Food Climate Research Unit at the University of Surrey (Food Climate Research Network, 2008) found that food produced in the UK accounts for 18.5 per cent of our total greenhouse gas emissions, with dairy and meat responsible for 8 per cent. The Food Climate Research Network report (2008) concludes that to hit greenhouse gas reduction targets we will have to cut our meat consumption. But this is an unpalatable proposition for a government that is also responsible for the economic welfare of farmers and is conscious of the nation's intolerance of already being preached to about alcohol misuse, smoking, diet and exercise. The government view is that telling people to stop eating meat as well will be a step too far. But according to public health campaigners, consumers should be encouraged to eat less red meat to improve their health and wellbeing. Our over-consumption of meat provides an example of how ecological public health links human and planetary wellbeing.

CONCLUSION

There is a wealth of scientific evidence that tracks the impact of food on mental and physical health and wellbeing. This chapter has shown how the development of national and local food policies has been influenced, or otherwise, by this evidence. In some areas, the evidence has been contested or ignored, such as, for example, around food and mental health and wellbeing issues. In other areas the linkages are well accepted. There is a disjuncture between evidence and public policy. It was the BSE crisis that forced the government to set up the FSA, whose initiatives to improve health and wellbeing have, in the view of public health campaigners, been adopted too slowly by the food industry. It appears that the coalition government wants to work far more closely with the food industry and is inviting food industry representatives onto committees designed to develop food policy. At the same time, in England, the FSA's responsibility for nutrition has been transferred to the DH, where policy can be better controlled by government.

Food is central to our wellbeing through food safety, food choices and the link between what we eat and our physical and mental health. At the same time, food is big business and there are powerful financial incentives for corporations to pursue practices that promote profit rather than health. The way government balances the interests of business with public health and the importance government gives to scientific evidence linking mental ill health and food will be a test of its commitment to the population's health and wellbeing in coming years.

Further reading and websites

Kayani, N. (2009) 'Food, health and wellbeing', in Stewart, J. and Cornish, Y. (eds) *Professional Practice in Public Health*. Exeter: Reflect Press Ltd

The Food Standards Agency, available at **www.food.gov.uk**

An independent agency to protect public health and consumer interests relating to food, with advice on food safety, nutrition and diet, and food protection.

Food Vision, available at **www.foodvision.gov.uk**

Case studies from around the country on how local government is promoting healthy eating and food safety.

Sustain, available at **www.sustainweb.org**

Sustain is the alliance for better food and farming advocating food and agriculture policies and practices that enhance the health and welfare of people and animals.

Chapter 9

Exercise and Wellbeing

Alfonso Jimenez, Silvano Zanuso and
Mark Goss-Sampson

Learning outcomes

In this chapter you will learn:

- the positive effects of exercise on wellbeing, based on the relevant evidence;

- the importance of an active lifestyle to improve wellbeing, health and quality of life;

- the potential reasons and actual hypotheses explaining why exercise provides a positive impact on wellbeing.

This chapter focuses on the positive effects of exercise in promoting wellbeing in the general population. The potential effects of exercise to influence general wellbeing and mental health are analysed, as well as the potential causes of those positive effects, based on the evidence.

INTRODUCTION

Participation in physical activity and exercise can result in desirable health outcomes in terms of both acute and chronic adaptations in the physiological and psychological domains (CDC, 1996). Physical activity, exercise, health and quality of life are closely interconnected. The human body is designed to move and therefore needs regular physical activity in order to function optimally and avoid illness. It has been proven that a sedentary lifestyle is a risk factor for the development of many chronic illnesses, including cardiovascular diseases that are a main cause of death in the Western world. Furthermore, living an active life brings many other social and psychological benefits, with a direct link between physical activity and life expectancy, so that physically active populations tend to live longer than inactive ones. Sedentary people who become more physically active report feeling better from both physical and mental points of view, and enjoy a better quality of life (European Commission, 2008).

The interest in the potential effect of physical activity and exercise on different aspects of mental health and general wellbeing is increasing. There is strong and consistent evidence, both from surveys and experimental studies, showing that physical activity and exercise make people feel better (Pedersen and Saltin, 2006). These effects are seen in populations of all ages and are independent of socioeconomic or health status. Furthermore, people who are aware of such benefits may be encouraged to increase commitment to regular exercise.

Notable among the mental health and wellbeing benefits are a reduction of anxiety and depression, decreased reactivity to psychological stress, and enhanced cognition. In this chapter we will discuss the positive impact of exercise on the first two areas, identifying the potential reasons for these effects and outlining the evidence for them.

POSITIVE EFFECTS OF EXERCISE RELATED TO WELLBEING: A SHORT UPDATE OF THE EVIDENCE

The effects of exercise in stress and anxiety reduction

As an example of the prevalence of stress and anxiety, it is estimated that work-related stress, depression or anxiety affected 415 000 individuals who had worked in the last 12 months in 2008/9 in the UK, with a corresponding estimated 11.4 million lost working days due to these work-related conditions. This represents an estimated average of 27.5 working days lost per affected case and makes stress, depression or anxiety the largest contributor to the overall estimated annual days lost from work-related ill health in 2008/9. The most common mental disorders were: mixed anxiety and depression (7 per cent for men, 11 per cent for women), anxiety (4 per cent for men, 5 per cent for women) and depression (2 per cent for men, 3 per cent for women). Worldwide lifetime prevalence of anxiety disorders is 16.6 per cent, with considerable heterogeneity between studies. In addition, most people experience episodic, and/or sometimes extended, stress-related symptoms during the course of their lives (Hatfield and Kaplan, 2004).

Regular physical activity and exercise has been reported to relieve the specific symptoms related with stress and anxiety (Petruzzello *et al.*, 1991). For many individuals, the alleviation of anxiety through exercise provides a strong stimulus for maintaining participation. According to a review of the literature by Landers and Arent (2001), in which they reviewed more than 100 scientific studies on the potential anxiety-reducing effect of exercise, small to moderate reductions in anxiety with exercise have been consistently reported in the exercise psychology literature over the last three decades, and especially in the mid-1990s (Calfas and Taylor, 1994; Kugler *et al.*, 1994; Landers and Petruzzello, 1994; Long and Van Stavel, 1995; McDonald and Hodgdon, 1991; Petruzzello *et al.*, 1991).

According to the recent review done by the US Physical Activity Guidelines Advisory Committee (CDC, 2008), the association between physical activity, exercise and reduced feelings of distress or enhanced wellbeing among adults was virtually unstudied in large groups of people before 1995. Since then, more than 30 population-based observational studies have been published, including nationally representative samples of more than 175 000 Americans. Most of the studies looked at cross-sectional associations, which indicated that active people on average had more than 30 per cent lower odds of feelings of distress or 30 per cent higher odds of enhanced wellbeing when compared with inactive people (CDC, 2008). These positive effects have been observed for aerobic forms of exercise across a wide range of intensities (cycling, walking, brisk walking, running, etc.), and for resistance exercise interventions based on low intensity and high volume (Bartholomew and Linder, 1998).

Antidepressive effects of exercise

Existing research evidence consistently shows that exercise impacts in a significant way in both men and women who are clinically classified as depressed, and for those experiencing transitory and/or less severe forms of depression, with stronger effects especially in the clinical population (North *et al.*, 1990; Craft and Landers, 1998). In this case, the monographic chapter about the mental health effects of physical activity and exercise of the Research Report of the US Physical Activity Guidelines (CDC, 2008) established that in more than 100 population-based observational studies published since 1995, active people on average had nearly 45 per cent lower odds of depression symptoms than did inactive people. In the national samples of Americans, active people had approximately 30 per cent lower odds of depression (CDC, 2008).

Therefore, considering that the general approach to the clinical treatment of depression is mainly based on psychiatric interventions, psychotherapy and drugs, exercise should now be considered as a core intervention for those individuals, based on the lack of unwanted side effects and its cost-effectiveness. In fact, exercise appears to be as effective as medication in people of both genders with clinical depression (Blumenthal *et al.*, 1999). At this point, and considering that many people experience episodic bouts of depression over stressful events in their lives, it seems that exercise offers a natural, appropriate and effective way to help them to cope and to feel better.

Subjective wellbeing, emotion and mood

A considerable number of studies on the effects of exercise on subjective wellbeing, emotion and mood have been published in recent decades. Biddle (2000) conducted a specific review and concluded that large-scale surveys in several countries using different methods and criteria confirm a moderate association between physical activity and indices of subjective wellbeing. Additionally, experimental studies support a positive effect on mood when utilising moderate intensity exercise.

Self-esteem and self-perception

Self-esteem is considered as an important indicator of emotional stability and adjustment, and therefore a construct of mental health. Focusing on this area, Fox (2000a, 2000b) reviewed 36 randomised controlled studies to establish the impact of exercise on self-esteem and found that only 50 per cent of those studies showed a positive effect. However, many of these studies applied either outdated or inappropriate instrumentation. Physical self-perceptions, including physical self-worth, body image, perceived competence and fitness are much more likely to show meaningful change through exercise than with other forms of intervention. There is clear evidence that exercise can change people's perceptions of their physical self and identity in a positive way. For some people, particularly those who are initially low in self-esteem, this may extend to more generalised changes in their perception of self.

Cognitive performance

In addition to the emotional or affective benefits, exercise appears to confer cognitive benefits as well. In fact, people who are physically fit seem to function more effectively than less physically active people on tasks involving intellectual demands (Hatfield and Kaplan, 2004). This kind of positive outcome seems to be particularly significant in older people (over 55 years of age) of both genders, who usually show some degree of decline on cognitive performance due to the natural ageing process (Sherwood and Selder, 1979).

Reviews by Boutcher (1999) and Etnier *et al.* (1997) focused on the impact of exercise on cognitive function (reaction time, memory, and fluid intelligence) in older people. Boutcher concluded that although cross-sectional studies show that fit older adults display better cognitive functioning than unfit older adults, the evidence from experimental studies remains equivocal. Etnier *et al.*'s meta-analysis, which focused on the relationship between fitness and cognitive performance in older adults, showed a weak but significant overall effect. It appears that the view that exercise into old age keeps you alert and sprightly has yet to be fully substantiated by additional research.

The impact of exercise on sleep quality

Insomnia affects approximately a third of the adult population and is associated with poor work performance and psychological dysfunction. Youngstedt *et al.* (1997) produced a meta-analysis of 38 studies on the effects of a single bout of exercise on the subsequent sleep of good sleepers. Exercise had no effect on the time it took to fall asleep, but did produce small increases in the amount of sleep time and SWS, and also reduced REM. This appears to be a fruitful area of research and the current limited evidence would suggest that exercise in bright light, with emphasis on duration rather than intensity, will improve sleep, regardless of usual sleep quality.

The negative effects of physical activity

In recent years news in the media regarding negative aspects of exercise and the concept of exercise addiction have created a kind of trend regarding the potential negative effects of exercise practice. Szabo (2000) addressed the literature to identify the potential existence of negative effects. He concluded that exercise dependence exists as a psychopathological disorder, but it is extremely rare. He suggested that exercise dependence is often confused with a high degree of exercise commitment, and outlined clear distinctions between the two, based on positive versus negative motivation and the degree of centrality of exercise in life. He cautioned that there are a significant number of people with eating disorders who use exercise to promote weight loss, but these can be distinguished from highly committed exercisers by their motivational profile. Female athletes, particularly those in sports where slenderness is required for performance and aesthetics, are at higher risk of developing eating disorders.

WHY IS EXERCISE GOOD FOR WELLBEING AND MENTAL HEALTH?

As already briefly discussed in this chapter, although an increasing amount of research in recent years has indicated that exercise is associated with improvements in mental health and wellbeing, a causal link has not been established and the underlying mechanism for this relationship remains unknown at this point (CDC, 2008). Based on current physiological and cognitive mechanisms, several hypotheses have been advanced as potential explanations for these positive effects of exercise on wellbeing.

The neurochemical hypothesis

Different studies in the past provided a number of plausible mechanisms through which exercise may improve mood and reduce symptoms of depression and anxiety. One of the earlier hypotheses implicated endogenous opioids, such as endorphins, in the mental health effects of exercise. Endorphins are chemical substances produced by the brain, pituitary glands and other body tissues, which act as natural opiates producing analgesia by binding to opiate receptor sites involved in perceptions of pain. More recently they have also been implicated in reward mechanisms and positive emotions (Raglin *et al.*, 2007). Physical stressors such as exercise can stimulate the production of endorphins, and this has led to the belief that endorphins are responsible for the popular perception that exercise makes you feel better after the practice.

The role and activities of other hormonal and physiological pathways have also been implicated in the possible positive benefits of exercise for wellbeing. An alternative hypothesis, based on the activity of different neurotransmitters, has been proposed. Neurotransmitters such as norepinephrine, dopamine and serotonin play a relevant role in depression disorders. It is believed that exercise may alter mood state through its effects on one or all of these neurotransmitters. The problem related to this hypothesis is the fact that most of the studies have been done with animals and, as concluded in a critical review included in *Exercise Psychology* by Buckworth and Dishman in 2002, this proposal, although suggestive, remains tentative until definitive studies can be done with humans.

The rhythmic nature of physical activity and exercise

The rhythmic nature of many forms of physical activity and exercise, such as walking, running or cycling at a steady pace for some time, helps to promote relaxation. This phenomenon has also been reported with other modes of exercise, such as exercise to music (for example, aerobics group exercise sessions) and those that require concentration on the quality of rhythmic movements (T'ai Chi).

This calming effect of rhythmic exercise may be biological, and it has been suggested that cerebral cortical arousal could be inhibited due to a volley of afferent rhythmic impulses from the muscles to an inhibitory or 'relaxation' site in the brainstem of the central nervous system (Bonvallet and Bloch, 1961; Hatfield, 1991; Meijer *et al.*, 2002).

The thermogenic effect of exercise

The model for the thermogenic effect of exercise is based mainly on animal studies (Von Euler and Soderberg, 1957). However, it appears that heat production during exercise represents a thermoregulatory inefficiency that produces a cascade of events leading to relaxation (Hatfield, 1991; Petruzzello *et al.*, 1991).

The hypothalamus detects any increase in the temperature of the body and consequently promotes a cortical relaxation effect. This results in decreased activation of motor neurons to the skeletal muscle fibres. In turn, the reduction in muscle efferent activity results in reduced muscle tension and a decrease in the sensitivity of the muscle spindles to stretch. This relaxation effect results in a concomitant reduction in sensory afferent feedback to the brainstem arousal centre, thus invoking a relaxed state (Hatfield and Kaplan, 2004).

Exercise as a social experience

An exercise session may provide a diversion or time-out experience from daily concerns and responsibilities that occupy the person's mind and that sometimes lead to stress. This is a clear 'change of mind' context, which is very attractive for most individuals. At the same time, and especially in social forms of exercise (team sports, group exercise practice, etc.), the social setting may involve meaningful social interaction that could alleviate stress and anxiety for everybody.

Commitment and success with the exercise goal

Commitment is a clear indicator of voluntary individual human behaviour. For any individual engaged in regular exercise practice, accomplishing the exercise goal may or may not alter how this person feels after exercise. When a person achieves their goals there is normally an associated positive sense of achievement. This change in psychological state resulting from exercise is referred to as the 'feel-better' phenomenon (Morgan, 1985) and is frequently reported by exercise practitioners as a proactive factor in promoting exercise adherence.

Case study 9.1 The Fit Age Project

A study, called the 'Better Ageing Study', supported by the European Community and involving eight universities in four countries – the UK, France, Belgium and Italy – was set up to investigate the benefits of physical activity on various health, physical and social aspects of a group of elderly Europeans. Part of this study was the 'Fit Age Study', the aim of which was to evaluate the effect of a 12-week strength training programme in a group of elderly participants, focusing on:

- dispositional anxiety;
- positive and negative effect;
- mood state profile.

The study involved a group of recreationally active elderly people of both genders (age range 65–80) living in the Manchester area who followed a 12-week strength training programme involving three training sessions per week.

Methods

Participants were divided into an immediate intervention group and a waiting list control group who trained subsequently. Strength performance, trait anxiety and POMS were measured in both groups at baseline and across 12 weeks.

Main results

- Training resulted in a statistically significant strength increase in the intervention group. Trait anxiety showed a decline in both groups.
- When mood profiles of participants were analysed across the initial 12 weeks of the study, the Vigour-Activity subscale of the POMS significantly decreased in the control group, while it remained at the pre-intervention level in the exercising group.
- The affect data showed that negative effect decreased significantly in the intervention group following 12 weeks of resistance training.

Conclusions

This study shows that increase in strength performance resulting from a 12-week period of resistance training in elderly individuals is associated with a significant reduction in negative effects. Further, positive aspects of mood states were maintained across the training period in the intervention group, while they declined in the waiting list control group.

Activity 9.1 Reflection

Considering the positive effects of exercise for wellbeing outlined in this chapter, write a basic rationale document (1 to 2 pages) on why people should be physically active. Be clear and concise, and provide some of the evidences of these positive effects.

CONCLUSION

To live an active life brings many social and psychological benefits and there is a direct link between physical activity and life expectancy, so that physically active populations tend to live longer than inactive ones. At the same time, sedentary people who become more physically active report feeling better from both physical and mental points of view, and enjoy a better quality of life.

Interest in the potential effect of physical activity and exercise on different aspects of mental health and general wellbeing is increasing. There is strong and consistent evidence, both from surveys and experimental studies, showing that physical activity and exercise make people feel better. These effects are seen in populations of all ages and are independent of socioeconomic or health status. Furthermore, people who are aware of such benefits may be encouraged to increase commitment to regular exercise.

However, although research in recent years has indicated that exercise is associated with improvements in mental health and wellbeing, a causal link has not been established and the underlying mechanism for this relationship remains unknown at this point.

Further reading and websites

www.health.gov/paguidelines

The website of the US Physical Activity Guidelines Advisory Committee (2008) has different materials for the general population, health and exercise professionals, health professionals, etc. On this website you can link directly to the *Physical Activity Guidelines Advisory Committee Report*, Chapter 8, which focuses on the benefits of exercise and physical activity for mental health and wellbeing.

www.euro.who.int/hepa

The website of the European Network for the Promotion of Health-Enhancing Physical Activity (HEPA Europe). On this site you can find information about intervention projects to promote physical activity and exercise, and the impact of these on health, wellbeing and quality of life.

www.exerciseismedicine.org

The website of the American College of Sports Medicine focuses on the impact of exercise as an effective tool for the prevention and treatment of chronic diseases related to lifestyle. You can find specific exercise intervention guidelines and different materials for health and exercise professionals, and health professionals (GPs, nurses, etc.).

Chapter 10

The Genetics and Genomics of Wellbeing

Harry Chummun

Learning outcomes

In this chapter you will learn how to:

- identify the relationship between genes, proteins and environment;

- elaborate on the significance of genetic (biological) markers influencing mood, happiness and subjective wellbeing;

- explain the contribution of genes in the promotion of health and wellbeing.

Wellbeing is a complex construct that concerns optimal experiences gained through growth and development for effective functioning within a given environment. The hedonic approach is concerned with happiness and defines wellbeing as attainment of pleasure and elimination or avoidance of pain, tissue damage and disease. The eudemonic approach focuses on the degree to which the person realises his full potential and addresses ideas of self-development, personal growth and purposeful engagement. These approaches function independently, but are often complementary to each other. Happiness and wellbeing may be affected by issues such as money, diet and environmental factors, but there is a growing acknowledgement that genetic and genomic factors are equally important in influencing healthy growth, development, happiness and life satisfaction.

INTRODUCTION

Genes are the main structures through which environmental factors and lifestyle influence health and wellbeing. Some genes carry codes for making proteins, while others (genomics) facilitate the transcription and the translation of these codes into proteins such as hormones, enzymes and neurotransmitters for cellular functions. Each inherited gene has unique codes and is the basis for individual variation. Based on the uniqueness of these proteins, an individual may have a healthy advantage over another, although genes are also responsible for ill health.

Such variations are also subject to environment damage (genetic mutation) due to conscious or unconscious effort on the part of the individual, producing abnormal proteins, altered organs and impaired functions. Abnormal proteins are often used as biomarkers to diagnose physical disorders such as cancers, as well as psychiatric disorders such as affective disorders and depression. While many proteins, and therefore genes, influence health and wellbeing, this chapter will identify the genes associated with the immune system, personality traits, exercise, serotonin, gender difference, obesity and age, and discusses their roles in the promotion of happiness, health and wellness.

Activity 10.1 Reflection

Inherited genes underpin health as well as disease.

1. Genes code, and genomics translate, genetic codes into proteins. Describe how genetic codes are transcribed into messenger ribonucleic acids (mRNAs) and how mRNAs are translated into proteins.
2. These proteins are selected from 21 human amino acids in a pool from ingested dietary proteins. Elaborate on the role the environment plays in producing these proteins.
3. Abnormal proteins cause disease. For example, faulty insulin causes diabetes mellitus. How can a person adapt his environment to reduce the symptoms of a genetic disorder? (Use phenylalanine (amino acid) from the diet in phenylketonuria (genetic disease) as an example.

THE GENETIC MECHANISM OF WELLBEING AND HEALTH

Darwin believed that certain behaviour patterns, including happiness and sadness, are genetically-based biological mechanisms that evolved as a survival mechanism. Facial expression of these basic emotions is universally recognised in all cultures, suggesting that they are a biological rather than a learnt response. Human infants display happiness and sadness, indicating distinct neurobiological mechanisms, and biological expression of these emotions may be aimed at key environmental foci to secure specific needs for self-fulfilment like, for example, the smiling infant pleases his mother in return for comfort (Darwin, 2007). Thus human ability to experience emotions has an evolutionary perspective; the presence of feelings designed to influence behaviour for self-actualisation is primarily recognised through physiological interactions with the environment.

GENES, HAPPINESS AND THE IMMUNE SYSTEM

Mood changes, such as loneliness, unhappiness and depression, have been linked to impaired immune system function. Happiness is known to lower blood pressure and stress hormones, and increase muscle flexion and immune function by raising infection-fighting T cells and B cells (O'Leary, 1990). Laughter increases several neurochemical syntheses, including interleukins (cytokines) that buffer the immunosuppressive effects of stress (Steptoe *et al.*, 2008). It triggers the release of pain-killing endorphins, and increases Complement 3 that helps antibodies to destroy infected cells (McGhee, 2010), as well as B- and T-cells, helper T cells and natural killer (NK) cells to protection against infections (Bennett *et al.*, 2003).

A genetic regulator (transcription factor progenitor cell), named Ctip2, differentiates and matures T cells from lymphocyte progenitor cells. Genetic mutation in this transcription factor results either in T cell depletion or in the production of immature T cells that do not protect against infections (Golonzhka *et al.*, 2007). Individuals with negative affective personalities, which lead to depression and low self-esteem, poorly recruit these immune system responses and are more at risk of infection than those who are positively affective. Depression may be associated with hypersecretion of several pro-inflammatory cytokines, including interleukin-5 (Leonard, 2000). Some cytokines are proteins, secreted by the immune system, which activate other immune system cells to induce 'stress-like' behavioural and neurochemical changes, supporting the hypothesis that hypersecretion of proinflammatory cytokines is involved in the pathology of mood-related ill health (Elenkov *et al.*, 2005).

GENES, PERSONALITY AND SUBJECTIVE WELLBEING

Is our ability to be happy solely dependent on individual lifestyle or is it constrained by personality? Personality is largely underpinned by our genes. Twin studies provide an experimental method to isolate the influence of genes, since identical (monozygotic) twins share 100 per cent of their genes. Identical behaviours will be due solely to their genetic make-up, even though being brought up in different environments can induce minor differences (nature vs. nurture). Weiss *et al.* (2008) investigated how monozygotic and non-identical (dizygotic) twins respond to openness, conscientiousness, extraversion, agreeableness and neuroticism, given that these emotions are linked to subjective wellbeing and overall feelings of happiness. Interviews with participants aimed to assess subjective wellbeing – the degree of satisfaction with, and control over, their own lives. The study showed that subjective wellbeing was negatively correlated with neuroticism, and positively correlated with extraversion, openness to experience, agreeableness and conscientiousness. The researchers concluded that, although happiness is subject to numerous external stimuli, 50 per cent of these traits are inherited, which can be explained by the genetic architecture of personality alone. For example, Gutknecht *et al.* (2007) demonstrated that mutations in the tryptophan hydroxylase-2 gene (TPH2), which codes for the rate-limiting enzyme serotonin (5-HT) in the brain and which modulates responses of limbic circuits to emotional stimuli, are linked to a spectrum of emotional dysregulations resulting in emotional instability and personality disorders, such as affective disorders.

GENES, EXERCISE AND WELLNESS

Regular exercise increases satisfaction, achievement and happiness, and reduces the incidence of disease, when compared with sedentary lifestyles (see also Chapters 9 and 11). This association appears to be non-causal and mediated by genetic factors that influence both the exercise behaviour and the feelings of general wellbeing (Stubbe *et al.*, 2007). In their study of 18–65 year-old monozygotes, dizygotes and related individuals, the association between leisure time exercise and life satisfaction and happiness was investigated. Exercise was noted to release endorphins (neurotransmitters) to alleviate pain and promote tissue healing. It also enhances positive mood and promotes neurogenesis in the hippocampus with an increase in learning ability and memory capacity (Van der Borght *et al.*, 2007). Exercise also increases expression of brain-derived neurotropic factor (BDNF) protein, which promotes neurogenesis to protect existing neurons from damage and improves the efficiency of existing neural signal transmission across the synapse clefts, further enhancing learning and memory (O'Leary, 2008). Furthermore, physically active people recover from mild depression more quickly, develop a more positive mental outlook and stay healthier longer than those who do not regularly exercise (Fox, 1999).

Exercise also increases levels of serotonin in the brain, which are low in people with mental depression (Mattson *et al.*, 2004). Serotonin has a reciprocal affinity for BDNF, boosting brain serotonin levels and vice versa, so exercise acts as a mood enhancer through the BDNF gene. Furthermore, when the body is subjected to painful stimuli, endorphins, released during exercise from the pituitary gland, block the transmission of pain signals, producing a euphoric feeling often associated with feelings of self-fulfilment. The euphoria may result from this pain-blocking process and the subsequent elevation of serotonin and dopamine in the brain (Nybo and Secher, 2004). Some individuals never attain such exercise-derived euphoria due to a rare genetic mutation in the cytochrome b gene, resulting in progressive exercise intolerance, proximal limb weakness and attacks of myoglobinuria (Andreu *et al.*, 1999).

GENES, SEROTONIN AND HEALTH

Serotonin is often regarded as the 'feel-good' chemical and has been implicated in the aetiology of depression (Murphy and Lesch, 2008). Serotonin is produced by neurons in the raphe nuclei of the brainstem, with axonal projections in the cerebral cortex, the amygdala, and in other brain regions. The availability and signalling potential of released serotonin, within the synapses, is regulated by the action of the serotonin re-uptake transporter (SERT or 5-HTT) in the pre-synaptic neurone, which captures serotonin molecules released into the synaptic cleft and transports them back into the pre-synaptic nerve terminal. The strength of serotonin activity in the serotonin receptors is inversely proportional to the number of functional serotonin transporter molecules present at the pre-synaptic membrane. This suggests that the more serotonin transporter receptors there are, the more serotonin will be removed from the cleft and will not be available to stimulate the post-synaptic nerve, thus reducing the strength of conduction of neural impulses across the synapse; this is necessary for smooth and effective communication among nerves (Canli and Lesch, 2007). Serotonin-selective re-uptake inhibitor (SSRIs) drugs, such as Fluoxetine (Prozac), block the reuptake of serotonin into nerve terminals through the serotonin transporter, thus reversing the putative deficit of serotonin function in depression (Sibille and Lewis, 2007).

Individuals inherit one 5-HTT gene from each parent. The healthy serotonin gene codes for a long protein and a mutation codes for a short protein. A promoter gene codes for a protein for initiating transcription and translation of the 5-HTT protein (see Figure 10.1).

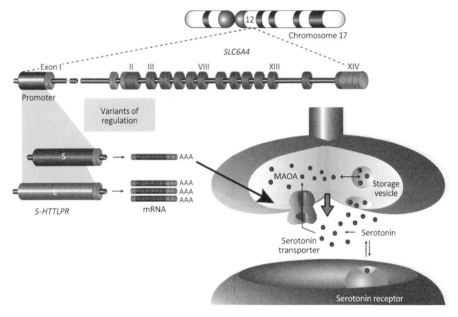

Figure 10.1 shows that the short (S) 5-HTTLPR variant of the 5-HTT gene (SLC6A4) produces significantly less 5-HTT mRNA and protein, as indicated by the arrow, than the long (L) variant, leading to higher concentrations of serotonin in the synaptic cleft. The short variant is associated with anxiety-related personality traits such as neuroticism, which are risk factors for affective spectrum disorders. MAOA = monoamine oxidase A

(Reprinted with permission from Macmillan Publishers Ltd: Canli, T. and Lesch, K. (2007) 'Long story short: the serotonin transporter in emotion regulation and social cognition'. *Nature Neuroscience*, 10: 1103–9.)

A mutation in this promoter gene has been shown to affect the rate of serotonin re-uptake due to lack of adequate 5-HTT and is linked to aggressive phenotype, post-traumatic stress disorder and depression (Canli and Lesch, 2007). The short allele is found in about half of

Caucasians, in whom even a single copy of the shortened 5-HTT gene causes stress-induced depression. This type of genetic disorder is not directly linked to depression *per se*, although it lowers the level of the transporter protein, which then leads to an increased experience of anxiety and distress and a gross exaggeration of mood changes, even with minimal changes in their relationships, jobs or financial situations (Nakamura *et al.*, 2000).

Serotonin has also recently been linked to social ranking theory, which suggests that a member who occupies a lower rank in an organisation or family setting often experiences increased unhappiness and depression. For example, the amount of food obtained for self or family consumption not only depends on the general availability of food but also on the person's ability to compete with others for this food. The 'stronger' the individual, the more food he obtains at the expense of the 'weaker' person. Larson and Summers (2001) proposed that serotonergic nerve activation is lower in the hippocampus, nucleus accumbens and brainstem of subordinate males but it is expressed more rapidly in dominant males. Furthermore, amygdalar serotonergic nerve activation also responds more rapidly in dominant males and more slowly in subordinate males. Thus people with elevated serotonin levels would display a more dominant behaviour in their environment at the expense of the less dominant people, even though their comparative output for the organisation may be similar. Social rank theory, therefore, argues that emotions and moods are significantly influenced by the perceptions of one's social status/rank; that is, the degree to which one feels inferior to others (Gilbert, 2008). Serotonin may be seen as not only influencing the perception of food availability but also of social rank.

Submissive behaviour is a common outcome of such perceptions, particularly in those at the lower end of a hierarchical structure. Feelings of failure, social anxiety and depression have been attributed to defensive submissive strategies leading to work-related stress, unhappiness, demotivation, frustration and anger (Allan and Gilbert, 2002). On the other hand, social feedback such as praise for jobs well done increases serotonin level, enhances self-esteem, raises individual expectations and drives self-actualisation.

GENES, GENDER DIFFERENCES AND WELLNESS

Gender appears to influence the perception of health, happiness and wellbeing due to differences in neurobiological responses, even though the biological structures are largely the same in both men and women.

Men, faced with a sad episode such as a very sick child, experience fewer mood disorders than women due to lower levels of biological responses in the male brain. Men activate a significantly smaller portion of their limbic system than women during transient sadness, indicating a clear difference in their brain chemistry and responses (Georgea *et al.*, 1996). The limbic system includes the amygdala, hippocampus and hypothalamus, connecting to various brain areas through neurones and neurotransmitters, and is mainly involved in motivation and emotional behaviours such as laughter and happiness. Women tend to be more expressive of love, happiness and sadness than males and have a better psychosocial adjustment to illness. Furthermore, women experience greater intensity, experience and frequency of both positive and negative affect, joy and love than men but also experience more embarrassment, guilt, shame, sadness, anger, fear and distress, placing them more at risk of unhappiness and depressive moods than men (Benyamini *et al.*, 2000). In addition, women are more prone to depression because of their tendency to dwell on the causes of negative emotions, whereas men distract themselves from dwelling on these emotions by using different cognitive strategies when faced with similar emotional situations (Hall *et al.*, 2000). These emotions and behaviours are partly the result of differences in the genetic make-up of men and women, which are responsible for the reduced levels of neurotransmitters such as dopamine, serotonin and norepinephrine in the brain circuitry (Kelly *et al.*, 1999).

GENES, AGE, HAPPINESS AND WELLNESS

Happiness is reported to be higher in the over-45 year-olds in the UK, leaving those below 45 as most vulnerable to being miserable and prone to depression (Blanchflower and Oswald, 2004). For both men and women the probability of unhappiness, lack of self-worth and depression peaks at around 44, irrespective of socioeconomic status, offspring, marital status or changes in jobs or income. It is proposed that older individuals learn to adapt to their strengths and weaknesses and, in mid-life, quell their unfeasible aspirations (Diener *et al.*, 2009). Hedonic wellbeing improves adaption to stress with a steady decline in experienced stress from age 22 onwards, reaching its lowest point at 85. Worry stays fairly steady until 50, then sharply tapers off, while anger decreases steadily from 18 and sadness rises to a peak by 50, then declines. Enjoyment and happiness are high in teenagers but, thereafter, decrease gradually until 50 but then rise steadily over the next 25 years (Blanchflower and Oswald, 2008). On the other hand, eudemonic wellbeing shows little variation by age from young adulthood through mid-life to old age. Personal growth, however, decreases across these age periods but it is unclear if these patterns are due to cohort differences or maturation processes (Kwan *et al.*, 2003). Such adaptation may possibly be due to environmental or/and psychological changes in the way older people view the world, or due to biological adaptation, for example in their brain chemistry or due to the local effects of endocrine changes (Stone *et al.*, 2010).

Pessimists and optimists

Pessimists have shorter telomeres than optimists (O'Donovan *et al.*, 2009). The telomeres are regions of deoxyribonucleic acids at the end of the chromosome that protect the genetic material in the chromosome from being lost each time the cell divides. Every time cells replicate, the chromosomes become a little shorter, but the enzyme telomerase helps rebuild telomeres to stave off this process. Telomerase levels naturally decline with age and this is often used as a biomarker for diagnosing the ageing process, as opposed to other diseases. Eventually the losses affect not only the telomeres but also the ability of the genes to keep on producing the proteins needed for effective cellular functions and health. Pessimistic individuals are unable to adapt very well to stress due to raised cortisol levels, which eventually damages the telomeres (Wolkowitz *et al.*, 2010). Levy *et al.* (2002) suggest that those who are more optimistic, happy and positive about getting older actually live longer and are happier than those who hold a pessimistic attitude about their own ageing. However, consumption of a balanced diet, based on sound nutritional education, adequate money and access to and availability of appropriate foods, reduces loss of telomeres. For example, eating a diet low in refined sugars and rich in fruits and vegetables, with only 10 per cent of calories derived from fat, and engaging in moderate aerobic exercise, relaxation techniques and breathing exercises, increases blood telomeres by 29 per cent and keeps us looking younger (Aubert and Lansdorp, 2008).

GENES, OBESITY AND WELLBEING

In the UK it is estimated that 20 per cent of men and 25 per cent of women are obese, and that as many as 30 000 people die prematurely from obesity-related diseases every year. At the current rate of increase, three-quarters of the UK population could be overweight, costing the National Health Service (NHS) £6.3 billion, by 2015 (McCormick and Stone, 2007). Personality traits such as neuroticism, obsessiveness and perfectionism are partially driven by genetics and have a role to play in some eating disorders such as anorexia nervosa and bulimia. Individuals with these personality features are often very anxious, depressed, perfectionists, self-critical and always striving to meet the highest standard of performance possible. They are often caught in a self-defeating cycle of fear and dissatisfaction when they fail to meet their expectations and goals. An increasing proportion of food consumption is driven by pleasure, not just for homeostatic needs.

For some people in affluent societies, the food environment creates a form of appetitive drive similar to that produced by other pleasure-driven activities such as compulsive gambling (Finlayson *et al.*, 1999). This phenomenon, known as hedonic hunger, is contributing to escalating obesity and its medical co-morbidities as the obese individuals prefer and consume more high-palatability foods than needed for normal weight and homeostatic needs. Among normal weight individuals, restrained eating behaviour may be attributed to diet-induced challenges to the homeostatic system, although this may be more likely to stem from hedonic hunger (i.e. eating less than wanted rather than less than needed), implying that obese individuals may be experiencing a compulsive behavioural eating disorder (Lowe and Butryn, 2007).

Aberrations in the biological mechanisms regulating normal eating behaviours have been linked to compulsive eating disorders. For example, pleasure-seeking behaviours, such as over-eating, could be due to disturbances in the neurological dopaminergic pathways, triggering a physical and emotional reaction to repeat that pleasure (Wang *et al.*, 2002). An abnormal tryptophan synthesis may be partially responsible for the disregulation of appetite, creating a sense of continuous hunger. Such eating behaviour disruption leads to depression and anxiety, both for under- and over-eaters, as well as other mental disorders such as obsessive compulsive disorder, bipolar disorder, borderline personality disorder and ADHD (Didonna, 2009).

Many genes contribute to compulsive eating disorders and obesity. Fat cells contain elevated concentrations of the enzyme lipoprotein lipase or low-density lipoproteins (LDL), whose synthesis is governed by genes. LDL enables fat cells to store triglycerides (fats), so the higher the concentration of LDL, the more easily cells store fat (Olson, 1998). Leptin is a protein hormone made by the ob (obese) gene inside fat cells to suppress appetite and accelerate metabolism. The brain cells of most obese people have a mutation in the leptin gene, keeping hunger at a very high level, resulting in over-eating and chronically raised body mass index (Jiang *et al.*, 2004). Fused toes and other abnormalities (FTO) is a gene on human chromosome 16 in which certain variants cause the production of an abnormal enzyme resulting in failure to regulate energy intake. This has also been linked to obesity in humans (Speakman *et al.*, 2008). These genes can also be inherited because co-occurrence of eating disorders such as compulsive over-eating among identical twins is greater than among fraternal twins, indicating a hereditary trend (Farooqi *et al.*, 1998).

Case study 10.1 Severe obesity in childhood

Scientists from the University of Cambridge and the Wellcome Trust Sanger Institute found duplication or deletion of large chunks of deoxyribonucleic acids from chromosome 16, called Copy Number Variants (CNVs), in some families with severe obesity from a young age. CNVs belong to the gene SH2B1, which is linked to obesity, autism and learning difficulties. Some of the 300 children in the study had been formally placed on the Social Services 'at risk' register, because it was suspected that the parents were deliberately over-feeding their children and causing their severe obesity. As a result of this study, they were removed from this register. Such evidence must alter attitudes and practices among health professionals responsible for the health and wellbeing of children at risk of obesity. Any remedial programme must include the full engagement of the patients or their carers.

CONCLUSION

Striving for happiness and general wellbeing, whether hedonic or eudemonic, is the lifetime pursuit of living organisms. Genetic factors account for substantial amounts of individual variation in achieving programmed wellbeing and health. Our ability to be happy and healthy is enhanced or impeded by the nature of the genes we inherit from our parents, as these genes set the parameters within which we function to achieve our predetermined level of happiness and self-actualisation. Genes are subject to change through our lifestyle and chemicals, e.g. drugs. With genetic variants, the proteins, such as hormones, neurotransmitters and those making up whole organs that are produced, will be altered and sub-optimal for homeostatic cellular functions. Then the body systems will be ill equipped to deal with the stressors of daily life and our ability to achieve happiness and wellbeing will be severely compromised. Health promoters must be aware of the genetic influence on health and wellbeing, and empower people to adopt healthier lifestyles in order to help their genome achieve optimum health and prevent ill health. However, while the health promoter has a duty of care, the individual is ultimately responsible for his/her own happiness and wellbeing.

Further reading and websites

GeneSense is available at **www.genesense.org.uk**

This is a case study-based educational site for health professionals and includes science, ethics and practice issues.

The Wellcome Trust is available at
www.wellcome.ac.uk

It provides general information on genetics, ethics and the Human Genome Project.

The British Society for Human Genetics is available at
www.bshg.org.uk

This is a professional organisation site representing UK human genetics professionals.

www.geneticseducation.nhs.uk

Develops materials and supports genetics education for health in the UK and worldwide.

Chapter 11

Promoting Wellbeing in Long-term Conditions

Silvano Zanuso and Alfonso Jimenez

Learning outcomes

In this chapter you will learn:

- the positive effects of physical activity and exercise on wellbeing in long-term chronic diseases patients, based on the relevant evidence;

- the importance of having an active lifestyle to improve wellbeing, health and quality of life for patients with long-term conditions.

This chapter focuses on the role of physical activity and exercise in promoting wellbeing in long-term conditions. The potential effects of physical activity and exercise to influence general wellbeing and mental health will be assessed. Various aspects of wellbeing will be analysed, with the aim of showing if the positive improvements in wellbeing observed in the general population can be identified in subjects with chronic conditions, with a specific focus on metabolic syndrome and type 2 diabetes based on the high prevalence of these disorders.

INTRODUCTION

Our modern way of living has largely eliminated physical activity as one of the fundamental stimuli of our lives. The growth of non-communicable lifestyle diseases and the epidemic increase in obesity provide clear evidence of this imbalance between our lifestyles and our physical requirements (European Commission, 2008).

Physical inactivity is a state of relatively complete physical rest, which does not provide sufficient stimulus for human organs to maintain their normal structures, functions and regulations. Physical inactivity has become a major risk factor for chronic non-communicable diseases in populations. Epidemiological research has proven that 15–20 per cent of the overall risk for coronary heart disease, type 2 diabetes, colon cancer, breast cancer and fractured hips in the elderly is attributable to physical inactivity. The overall disease burden in the European Region caused by physical inactivity is estimated to be 3.5 per cent (European Commission, 2008). In 2008, almost a quarter of adults (24 per cent of men and 25 per cent of women aged 16 or over) in England were classified as obese (BMI 30 kg/m^2 or over), and a greater proportion of men than women (42 per cent compared with 32 per cent) were classified as overweight (BMI 25 to less than $30kg/m^2$). At the same time, 39 per cent of adults had a raised waist circumference in 2008 compared to 23 per cent in 1993. Women were more likely than men (44 per cent and 34 per cent respectively) to have a raised waist circumference (over 88 cm for women and over 102 cm for men). Both overweight and obesity are characterised by the accumulation of excessive levels of body fat and contribute to heart disease, hypertension, diabetes and some cancers, as well as psychosocial and economic difficulties. The cost of treatment of weight reduction is now estimated to exceed $117 billion annually in the USA. In the UK the direct cost of obesity to the NHS is £0.5 billion, while the indirect cost to the UK economy is at least £2 billion. By 2015, the *Foresight Report* (UK Government Office for Science, 2007) estimates that 36 per cent of males and 28 per cent of females (aged between 21 and 60) will be obese. By 2025 it is estimated that 47 per cent of men and 36 per cent of women will be obese.

As has been discussed in Chapter 9, the available evidence from observational, prospective cohort studies, which are summarised in the latest *Physical Activity Guidelines Advisory Committee Report* (2008), supports the conclusion that physical activity and exercise have protective benefits for several aspects of physical, mental health and general wellbeing. There is strong evidence for protection against all the chronic pathologies, as well as for symptoms of the major mental disorders: depression and cognitive decline, anxiety and poor sleep, feelings of distress and fatigue (Pedersen and Saltin, 2006). Thus, current evidence supports the conclusion that regular participation in moderate to vigorous physical activity, consistent with current public health guidelines, confers physical and mental health benefits when compared to participation in low levels of physical activity or a sedentary lifestyle (CDC, 2008).

Since the publication of the Surgeon General's report on *Physical Activity and Health* (1996), the following definitions are utilised worldwide in the context of exercise science:

- **Physical activity**: bodily movement produced by the contraction of skeletal muscle that requires energy expenditure in excess of resting energy expenditure.
- **Exercise**: a subset of physical activity: planned, structured and repetitive bodily movement performed to improve or maintain one or more components of physical fitness.
- **Physical fitness**: this includes cardio-respiratory fitness, muscular fitness and flexibility.

However, considering that in the studies analysing the effects of physical activity and exercise on quality of life and general wellbeing those terms are not always operationally well defined, in this chapter the terms 'physical activity' and 'exercise' will be used interchangeably.

PHYSICAL ACTIVITY, EXERCISE AND WELLBEING IN LONG-TERM CONDITIONS

A physically active lifestyle is important for the prevention and treatment of many chronic diseases and conditions. Although the case for exercise has largely been built around its impact on physical health, including a positive impact on both the prevention (Pan *et al.*, 1997; Ramachandran *et al.*, 2006; Tuomilehto *et al.* 2001) and the management of chronic conditions as summarised in the *Physical Activity Guidelines Advisory Committee Report* (2008) and in the American Diabetes Association technical review (Sigal *et al.*, 2004), there is a growing interest in its potential to influence mental health and general wellbeing. In fact, the dimensions of health (physical, mental, emotional, social, etc.) are not separate from each other. For example, mental health problems are often interrelated with physical health problems such as coronary heart disease, cancer, diabetes, obesity, coronary obstructive pulmonary disease, HIV, neurological disorders and back pain (Steptoe, 2006).

General wellbeing and quality of life are frequently measured in investigations involving both clinical and general populations. As has been extensively discussed in Chapter 9, in the general population there is strong and consistent evidence, mainly from surveys, showing that physical activity makes people feel better, as well as feeling better about themselves, and feeling happier and more satisfied with life (Biddle *et al.*, 2000). These positive effects are independent of age and socioeconomic status. Based on the published evidence, successful treatment for chronic conditions encompasses multiple dimensions of health, including physical, functional, social and psychological wellbeing. It is generally accepted that physical activity participation may be associated with the improvement of general wellbeing and quality of life. However, the association of physical activity and improvements of general wellbeing and quality of life has not received the same level of interest in subjects with chronic conditions as compared with the general population (Zanuso *et al.*, 2009).

Exercise counselling for individuals with long-term conditions

The first step to increase quality of life through physical activity and/ or exercise is to motivate the subjects to change their physical activity habits, and this is an aspect that has been largely addressed in the literature. In fact, patients with chronic conditions can be motivated to become active, and exercise counselling delivered by exercise specialists seems to be an effective modality. A 30-minute one-to-one discussion based on the transtheoretical model of stages of change (Marcus and Simkin, 1994) delivered by a trained exercise specialist, and designed to educate, strengthen motivation and develop realistic strategies to promote physical activity, was found to be superior to standard exercise leaflets (Kirk *et al.*, 2001).

Additionally, the role of exercise counselling was investigated in numerous studies (Di Loreto *et al.*, 2005; Kirk *et al.*, 2004; Tudor-Locke *et al.*, 2004) and all reported the effectiveness of this form of intervention in clinical or wellbeing parameters. Interestingly, in a study published by Praet *et al.* (2008) it was shown that the prescription of group-based brisk walking represented an equally effective intervention to modulate glycemic control and cardiovascular risk profile in type 2 diabetes patients when compared with more individualised medical fitness programmes.

Exercise counselling has the objective of increasing readiness and motivation towards physical activity. These goals can be achieved by applying existing models, such as the transtheoretical model (Marcus and Simkin,1994; Tudor-Locke *et al.*, 2002; Tudor-Locke *et al.*, 2004) or by developing new counselling approaches (Di Loreto *et al.*, 2005). The effects of counselling interventions have been evaluated more in relation to health rather than to psychological outcomes. However, some available evidence suggests that some wellbeing-related parameters can also benefit from physical activity.

Physical activity and exercise interventions for individuals with long-term conditions

Exercise and congestive heart failure

In regard to long-term conditions (clinical populations), the area that has been extensively investigated is related to heart failure. Patients with congestive heart failure (CHF) show evidence of anxiety and depression, and experience a dramatic reduction in their quality of life. Clinical trials in those patients have shown that increasing exercise capacity can lead to significant improvements in quality of life. The evidence therefore suggests that exercise can play an important role in improving the function and quality of life in CHF patients (Lloyd-Williams and Mair, 2005).

Exercise and obesity

In addition, if we briefly review the impact of physical activity and exercise on the wellbeing of obese patients, the research shows that obesity and exercise are related to subjective wellbeing. In fact, many overweight individuals have low levels of subjective wellbeing as a reflection of 'anti-fat' biases and sociocultural considerations (Berger, 2004). Since exercise helps balance the energy intake–output equation and is associated with mood benefits, improved self-concept and self-esteem, and decreased stress levels, it seems to be an ideal approach for interrupting the inactivity–obesity cycle. Berger (2004) concludes that it is important that exercise is enjoyed, as this influences the psychological benefits of physical activity and exercise adherence in overweight and obese individuals.

A randomised control trial (Nieman et al., 2000) studied the effects of 12 weeks of exercise training (five 45-minute walking sessions per week at 60 per cent to 75 per cent maximum heart rate) and/or moderate energy restriction (1200 to 1300 kcal per day) on the psychological general wellbeing and profile of mood states in obese women. General wellbeing was improved, especially in four of six subscales: freedom from health concern or worry; life satisfaction; cheerful versus depressed mood; and relaxed versus tense feelings.

Exercise and diabetes

Dimensions of general wellbeing and quality of life were also studied in diabetic patients. In a relevant study (Hirsch et al., 2000) it was found that a single questionnaire did not cover all relevant aspects of the quality of life of subjects with type 2 diabetes. Thus, quality of life in diabetic people should be evaluated with different scales. In another study (Goldney *et al.*, 2004), the prevalence of depression in the diabetic population was found to be 24 per cent compared with 17 per cent in the non-diabetic population. A supplementary analysis comparing both depressed diabetic and depressed non-diabetic groups showed that there were statistically significant differences in the quality-of-life effects between the two depressed populations.

In the aforementioned studies the effects of exercise were measured on the dimensions constituting the core of subjective wellbeing: physical and social functioning; emotion and moods; self-esteem and self-perception; cognitive performance; and sleep quality.

Metabolic syndrome-related studies

Considering that usually an individual is affected by several chronic conditions at the same time, the metabolic syndrome is probably the condition that best represents a typical patient suffering from a long-term pathology. The metabolic syndrome (IDF, 2005) is a cluster of different metabolic risk factors (for example, impaired glucose tolerance, insulin resistance, high blood pressure, altered lipid profile). We will therefore focus on studies encompassing these metabolic risk factors, which seem to be directly linked to the development of atherosclerotic cardiovascular disease and to an increase in the risk of developing type 2 diabetes mellitus.

The Diabetes Prevention Program Study Group, which conducted one of the major randomised clinical trials analysing the efficacy of intensive lifestyle, metformin and placebo in the prevention of type 2 diabetes in people with impaired glucose tolerance (DPP Research Group, 2004), published a number of articles on different aspects of their study. One of these related studies was focused on the psychological domain (Delahanty *et al.*, 2002). However, in this study they did not evaluate the effects of intensive lifestyle on aspects of wellbeing, rather they evaluated how psychological and behavioural variables correlated with baseline body mass index (BMI). The authors found that lower exercise efficacy, lower weight loss, low fat diet self-efficacy, higher perceived stress, emotional eating, poor dietary restraint and binge-eating frequency and severity all correlated with higher baseline BMI.

Toobert *et al.* (2003), applying a comprehensive lifestyle self-management programme comprising a Mediterranean low saturated-fat diet, stress-management training, exercise, group support and smoking cessation, showed that postmenopausal women with metabolic syndrome can make comprehensive lifestyle changes that may lead to significant improvement both in clinical and quality of life parameters.

In another interesting study, published by Rejesky *et al.* (2006), a series of relevant correlates of health-related quality of life were examined in 5145 overweight or obese persons with type 2 diabetes, using the SF-36 and the Beck Depression Inventory. Analyses examined the potential relationship of demographic characteristics, disease burden and cardiovascular fitness to health-related quality of life. Interestingly, less desirable physical component scores (PCS) of the SF-36 were related also to low metabolic equivalent (aerobic capacity). Interactions between categories of obesity and aerobic capacity revealed that greater BMI was related to lower PCS when individuals had lower aerobic capacities, whereas in fact it was absent for those individuals who had higher aerobic capacities. In addition, although greater BMI was associated with more severe depressive symptomatology, this association was the most dramatic for those with class III obesity who had low aerobic capacity. More importantly, the interactions between obesity class and aerobic capacity suggested that the adverse effect of BMI may be buffered by higher aerobic capacities.

Ménard *et al.* (2007) studied a group of poorly controlled blood glucose subjects ($HbA_{1c} \geq 8$ per cent) and demonstrated that quality of life improved significantly despite the inherent constraints imposed by intensive multitherapy, comprising monthly clinical and biochemical assessment education sessions on diet and physical exercise.

Colberg *et al.* (2008), using two cognitive tests (Mini-Mental State exam, and the Saint Louis University Mental Status exam), have shown that some types of physical activity, including light and moderate exercise, appear to be beneficial to mental function in individuals with metabolic syndrome. In this case-control study it was shown that having diabetes, particularly when less well controlled, is associated with lower cognitive function scores, and physical activity participation may prevent some of the potential decline in cognition.

Case Study 11.1 The effects of exercise training on older patients with major depression

Background

Previous observational and interventional studies have suggested that regular physical exercise may be associated with reduced symptoms of depression. However, the extent to which exercise training may reduce depressive symptoms in older patients with major depressive disorder (MDD) has not been systematically evaluated.

Objective

To assess the effectiveness of an aerobic exercise program compared with standard medication (i.e. antidepressants) for treatment of MDD in older patients, we conducted a 16-week randomised control trial.

Methods

One hundred and fifty-six men and women with MDD (age ≥50 years) were assigned randomly to a program of aerobic exercise, antidepressants (sertraline hydrochloride) or combined exercise and medication. Subjects underwent comprehensive evaluations of depression, including the presence and severity of MDD, using the *Diagnostic and Statistical Manual of Mental Disorders* (4th Ed.) criteria, the Hamilton Rating Scale for Depression (HAM-D) and the Beck Depression Inventory (BDI) scores before and after treatment. Secondary outcome measures included aerobic capacity, life satisfaction, self-esteem, anxiety and dysfunctional cognitions.

Results

After 16 weeks of treatment, the groups did not differ statistically on HAM-D or BDI scores (P = .67); adjustment for baseline levels of depression yielded an essentially identical result. Growth curve models revealed that all groups exhibited statistically and clinically significant reductions on HAM-D and BDI scores. However, patients receiving medication alone exhibited the fastest initial response; among patients receiving combination therapy, those with less severe depressive symptoms initially showed a more rapid response than those with initially more severe depressive symptoms.

Conclusions

An exercise training program may be considered an alternative to antidepressants for treatment of depression in older persons. Although antidepressants may facilitate a more rapid initial therapeutic response than exercise, after 16 weeks of treatment exercise was equally effective in reducing depression among patients with MDD.

Blumenthal, J.A., Babyak, M.A., Moore, K.A., Craighead, W.E., Herman, S., Khatri, P., Waugh, R., Napolitano, M.A., Forman, L.M., Appelbaum, M., Doraiswamy, P.M., Krishnan, K.R. (1999) *Arch Intern Med*, 159: 2349–56.

Case Study 11.2 Changes in cardio-respiratory fitness, psychological wellbeing, quality of life and vocational status following a 12-month cardiac exercise rehabilitation programme

Aim

To examine and evaluate improvements in cardio-respiratory fitness, psychological wellbeing, quality of life and vocational status in post-myocardial infarction patients during and after a comprehensive 12-month exercise rehabilitation programme.

Subjects

The sample population comprised 124 patients with a clinical diagnosis of myocardial infarction (122 men and two women).

Interventions

Sixty-two patients were randomly allocated to a regular weekly aerobic training programme, three times a week for 12 months, and were compared with 62 matched controls who did not receive any formal exercise training. A five-year follow-up questionnaire/interview was subsequently conducted on this population to determine selected vocational/lifestyle changes.

Results

Significant improvements in cardio-respiratory fitness ($p < 0.01$–0.001), psychological profiles ($p < 0.05$–0.001) and quality of life scores ($p < 0.001$) were recorded in the treatment population when compared with their matched controls. Although there were no significant differences in mortality, a larger percentage of the regular exercisers resumed fulltime employment and they returned to work earlier than the controls. Controls took lighter jobs, lost more time from work, and suffered more non-fatal reinfarctions ($p < 0.05$–0.01).

Conclusions

Regular supervised and prolonged aerobic exercise training improves cardio-respiratory fitness, psychological status and quality of life. The trained population also had a reduction in morbidity following myocardial infarction, and significant improvement in vocational status over a five-year follow-up period.

Dugmore, L. *et al.* Action Heart, Cardiac Rehabilitation Centre, Wellesley House, 117 Wellington Road, Dudley, West Midlands DY1 1UB, UK. Published in *Heart*, April 1999; 81(4): 359–66.

Activity 11.1 Reflection

Considering some of the effects of physical activity and exercise for wellbeing in patients with long-term conditions analysed in this chapter, discuss the potential impact of this action (to start an exercise programme) on the quality of life of those patients. Try to be clear and concise, but provide some of the evidence of the positive effects.

CONCLUSION

Physical activity and exercise promotion is an excellent public health intervention because of its positive effects on various chronic medical conditions, physical and mental function, and quality of life.

The interest in the potential effect of physical activity and exercise on different aspects of mental health and general wellbeing is increasing. There is strong and consistent evidence both from surveys and experimental studies showing that physical activity makes people feel better. These effects are seen in populations of all ages and are independent of socioeconomic or health status. Physical activity helps people feel better by reducing state and trait anxiety and improving mood. It can also help people feel better about themselves through improvements in physical self-perception and self-esteem, particularly in those with initial low self-esteem. Physical activity can also help reduce physiological reactions to stress and it may also improve sleep quality. Thus, the dimensions of wellbeing that can be improved with physical activity are: physical and social functioning; subjective wellbeing; emotion and moods; self-esteem and self-perception; cognitive performance; and sleep quality.

Wellbeing improvements through physical activity were investigated less frequently in the clinical populations than in healthy subjects. The area related to heart failure has been more extensively investigated than other clinical populations. The evidence suggests that exercise can play an important role in improving the function and quality of life with CHF patients.

Additionally, the effects of exercise on wellbeing were analysed in a number of studies involving patients with obesity, diabetes and the metabolic syndrome. A significant effort was made to evaluate the efficacy of exercise counselling, but unfortunately the outcomes were often measured only in terms of physiological parameters. Nevertheless, a significant amount of literature has analysed the benefits of physical activity on wellbeing and reports positive effects but, to our knowledge, there are no systematic reviews or meta-analyses that have been carried out to evaluate the effect of physical activity on wellbeing in this particular class of patients.

Further reading and websites

www.acsm.org
Website of the American College of Sports Medicine, the world-leading organisation in physical activity and exercise related to health. The most interesting contents focused on long-term conditions are a group of review documents called 'Position Stands', which summarise the actual evidence published about the positive impact of physical activity and exercise in specific long-term conditions.

www.exerciseismedicine.org
Another website of the American College of Sports Medicine focused on the impact of exercise as an effective tool for the prevention and treatment of chronic diseases related to lifestyle. You can also find specific exercise intervention guidelines and different materials for health and exercise professionals and health professionals (GPs, nurses, etc.).

www.health.gov/paguidelines

Website of the US Physical Activity Guidelines (2008), with different materials for the general population, health and exercise professionals, health professionals, etc. On this website you can directly access the *Physical Activity Guidelines Advisory Committee Report*, Chapter 8, which is focused on the benefits of exercise and physical activity for mental health and wellbeing, with some concrete references to long-term conditions.

www.euro.who.int/hepa

The website of the European Network for the Promotion of Health-Enhancing Physical Activity (HEPA Europe). On this site you can find information about intervention projects to promote physical activity and exercise, and the impact of these on health, wellbeing and quality of life.

Part 4: Social Approaches to Wellbeing

Chapter 12

Social Policy and Wellbeing
Allan McNaught and Simten Malhan

Learning outcomes

In this chapter you will learn how to:

- understand the role of public policy in modern society;

- identify the values and assumptions that underlie social policy in post-industrial society;

- assess how far 'wellbeing' has influenced contemporary social policy in the UK and Turkey.

But not all men are in this sense ordinary. As the means of information and of power are centralised, some men come to occupy positions in American society from which they can look down upon, so to speak, and by their decisions mightily affect the everyday worlds of ordinary men and women. They are not made by their jobs; they set down and break down jobs for thousands of others; they are not confined by simple family responsibilities; they can escape ... whether or not they profess their power, their technical and political experience of it far transcends that of the underlying population. (Wright-Mills, 1962, p. 3)

The concept of wellbeing is complex and involves many fundamental questions about the ordering of society, access to resources, and the value placed on the lives and wellbeing of others. These issues are political and the judgements made about them inform both public and social policy broadly, as well as informing particular social policies. This chapter provides an overview and analysis of public and social policy making and attempts to locate the influence of wellbeing in contemporary social policy in the UK, with some comparisons with Turkey.

INTRODUCTION

Public policy analyses and explores the nature of policy choices, their implementation and management. A sister discipline is public administration, the area that studies the theory and practice of the administration of the state and state agencies. There is overlap between public policy and public administration, while social policy, its implementation and management, is a subfield that crosses both these disciplinary areas.

The term 'policy' is often used to describe a domain or sphere of activity that is marked by decisions that share certain characteristics or focus. 'Social policy' refers to that domain of decisions that concern social welfare matters within a society. These range from the provision of goods and services, through to income maintenance measures, as well as legislation to protect the vulnerable or to promote particular values, or behaviour change on the part of individuals, communities and organisations. This use of the term 'social policy' is purely descriptive: it does not concern the content or the substance of the actual policies.

EXPLORING THE POLICY PROCESS

'Policy' is used to describe decision making that is characterised by a certain level of generality. 'Policies limit an area within which a decision is to be made and ensure that the decision will be consistent with and contribute to an objective' (Koontz *et al.*, 1982, p. 67). For Starling, policies are 'laws that are in scope and impact major attempts to solve problems or to seize opportunities' (Starling, 1982, p. 27).

There is another strand of the literature that is normative in its orientation, in that it describes how a policy or a decision should be made. This 'classical' approach to policy making sees it occurring in a stepwise fashion. This normally starts with the definition of a problem; gathering data about its characteristics and magnitude; developing options to solve the problem; and then choosing the most appropriate or suitable option. Variously called the linear, mainstream, common-sense or rational model, this model is the most widely held view of the way in which policy decisions are made. It suggests that policy making is a problem-solving process: rational, balanced, objective and analytical. In the model, decisions are made in a series of sequential phases, starting with the identification of a problem or issue and ending with a set of activities to solve or deal with the problem or issue (Sutton, 1999).

This depiction of policy making by individuals and organisations motivated many researchers and thinkers to look at the process critically and to test its underlying assumptions of rationality and comprehensiveness. The initial questioning focused on the notion of rationality, with writers like Herbert Simon (1957) and Charles Lindblom (1979) advancing explanative theories, which took account of the intellectual, resource and personal limitations of real people in real organisations. Simon saw decision makers as actors responding to the stimulus of dissatisfaction, often having several conflicting goals, with a limited ability to perceive and understand the environment. On the other hand, Lindblom describes the decision-making process as more characterised by 'muddling through' rather than by rational processes.

Both Simon and Lindblom identify the complex nature of decision making and the many interactions that are necessary for it to take place. Lindblom was particularly concerned about the constraints imposed by existing decisions and the framework of ongoing policy processes. He argued that the definition of a problem was itself a decision to be taken. Other critics of the rational model, such as Elmore, also suggest certain techniques, like 'backward mapping', which they believe would improve the decision-making process (Elmore, 1979).

These descriptions of how policies or decisions are made are but one facet of at least three spheres in which the concept of policy making can be explored. Firstly, there is that sphere that involves politicians, political ideologies and processes. These ideologies and political agendas set out expectations of what the state should do and be responsible for. The second sphere of action concerns activities in the bureaucratic organisations that serve politicians to provide advice and deliver the policies for which the politicians have a mandate. The third sphere is the settings and organisations in and through which policy is actually delivered or implemented.

Politics and the role of the state are therefore integral components of policy, and it rests on the notion that it is legitimate for the state to intervene in society to promote social objectives. This modern conception of the role of the state is widely attributed to Keynesian economics that urged state action to promote social and economic stability. There are variations on this theme across modern political philosophies. On the one hand, the liberal-democratic free-market state facilitates and regulates the market, providing a safety net for those who fail or are unable to compete. Then there are the 'centrist' notions of the state, where the state owns some of the means of production or operates in a 'corporatist' fashion. A more recent paradigm of the role of the state being advanced in political economy is the model of the 'competition state', one that tries to operate at a strategic level and through state agencies based on notions of (economic) efficiency and effectiveness. This is seen as a necessary process to make the country itself more regionally and globally competitive, and attractive to foreign direct investment.

THE ROLE OF THE STATE AND STATE POWER IN POLICY

Theories of policy and implementation highlight the importance of both the formal and informal elements of the exercise of political power and policy making in a state. They suggest that certain areas are regarded as 'high policy'. These areas are concerned with the fundamental existence of a state. These are invariably economic, foreign affairs and defence policies. Other matters are generally seen as 'low policy' although, under certain circumstances, these can be elevated to 'high policy' status. For any policy researcher a starting point for enquiry must include any statements of formal, informal or observed policy or priority for the particular area about which they are concerned. Politicians give priority to areas for a mixture of personal, political and situational reasons. To understand power, you also need to know and understand the process through which power is exercised (Walt, 1994). Generic theories give us that understanding by providing a variety of concepts to describe and analyse the nature and structure of power, as well as how it is exercised within political, organisational and social structures, and by groups and individuals.

In most countries it is government bureaucracies that work in support of politicians to formulate, promulgate and implement public policy. At this level in the political system, policy formulation involves the framing of legislation and associated regulations. It also involves making choices about how a policy should be implemented and the drawing up of timetables and schedules to roll out the policy. Some bureaucracies also implement policies directly or through their field offices. This strategic and implementation/management component of policy makes it important to have an understanding of how government bureaucracies function.

Understanding bureaucracies is also important for assessing what happens in large private and non-governmental organisations, because the bureaucratic form of organisation has been taken as a generic model for organisation and management in the modern world. Simon sees bureaucracies as 'the most effective tools that we humans have found for meeting human needs' (Simon, 1957).

Traditional political and public administration theories have been descriptive and formalistic. They located power in structures, attached to the formal offices, whether elected or appointed, and in the legal structure. Notions of power, influence and the policy process as critical components of how policy is made and implemented within bureaucracies only came to the fore in the early 1920s, when a series of 'community power studies' was undertaken with the simple objective of determining 'who governs'? They sought to identify what persons and which groups decided the fate of a community, whether through control of the formal power structure or through informally exercised influence (Lynd and Morrell, 1929, 1937). Within bureaucratic organisations, the notion of power has also evolved from positional or structural notions to those that incorporate more complex patterns of organisational behaviour.

The formal or structural notions of power in organisations are covered in the approach taken by Weber. His concept was that 'offices are arranged hierarchically, the rights of control and complaint between them being specified' (Albrow, 1977, p. 43). More specifically, his assumption was that the 'higher' the post, the greater the power exercised by individual office holders. This is the situation commonly depicted by organisation charts.

Activity 12.1

Identify a local wellbeing initiative or policy that has been adopted in your area by a health or local authority. All public authority minutes and papers are now in the public domain. Using these public sources, attempt to identify the following:

- What evidence was considered to justify the project or initiative?
- Who was the driving force behind the initiative? Was it the community, politicians, professionals or a coalition of some or all of these (and other) actors?
- How do you explain why the project or initiative was adopted?

WELLBEING AND PUBLIC POLICY IN TURKEY

'Transformation in Health' is the name of the health reform programme initiated by the Ministry of Health in Turkey in 2003. The aim of these reforms was to provide access to health care services for all, offering them fairly and equally to all citizens, and also increasing the quality of life through effective, efficient and fair health care services.

Effectiveness was a key underlying aim for increasing the health quality and level of health care services for the people. This included physical health and also the improvement of environmental, social and mental wellbeing. Preventive medicine and health care services have been strengthened. Of particular note has been a scheme to keep track of health outputs through evaluation and assessment. This has been facilitated by the introduction of a comprehensive health care registration system called 'Medula' covering all Turkish citizens.

Another aim of this reform programme was to ensure citizens' access to health care services and the elimination of the discrepancies between the regions of Turkey, thereby doing away with the differences between health indicators and wellbeing. Owing to the inequality between urban and rural areas and also different levels of health care services in the eastern and western regions of the country, a vertical organisational structure has been implemented. This has led to dramatic improvements in primary health care services. The sharing of responsibilities in health care services and introducing a 'single source of finance' system for each patient can be counted as the major factors leading to the success of the reforms. Therefore, the citizen's preferred physician carries out individual preventive measures and primary diagnostic and treatment services.

The reform programme has involved a reshaping of the Turkish Ministry of Health (MOH), whose primary role is now to regulate the health sector and shape policies concerning health matters. The priorities of the MOH are to determine the efficient, effective and fair use of resources.

A restructured compulsory general health insurance covering the whole society has been in operation since 2008. Through this scheme citizens contribute insurance premiums and make use of health care services as needed. The previous system was fragmented, offered different levels of benefits and was marred by deficits. The discrepancy in the level of health care services offered previously gave rise to injustice among citizens.

The new system has created a friendly atmosphere between the physician and citizen and has helped in enabling the former to assume an important role in health education, preventive medicine and general improvement in health. Over the past two years there has been a considerable decline in the amount of medical equipment and medicines wasted, which had previously constituted the greatest proportion of overall medical expenditure in Turkey. The establishment of trust between primary care physicians and patients has also been the key in enabling Turkey to set up an effective referral system for secondary and tertiary care.

All the hospitals in Turkey, whether state or private, render service to all citizens on condition that they enter into an agreement with the general health insurance and comply with the referral system regulations. In financing health care, it is not the institutions but the individuals that are given support. The institutions – or enterprises – that offer health care services are paid in proportion to the service they offer.

The fundamental objective of Turkey's health reforms is to help improve the health care system, protect and improve public health and increase the level of wellbeing across the society. This example shows the role of health policy and the linkage between health and wellbeing.

WELLBEING AND PUBLIC POLICY IN THE UK

Wellbeing has entered UK social policy discourses through its linkage with health, and was seen as a predominantly subjective phenomenon. This development has been perceived as part of a global convergence of the terms health and wellbeing. (Ganesh and McAllum, 2010.)

The root to this development lies in a long-standing recognition, by academics and the public, of the limitations of modern medicine. Illich (2001), first published in 1975, launched a trenchant attack on the medical establishment, which he regarded as a major threat to health. The dysfunctions of medicine that he identified included iatrogenic diseases, the impotence of the medical services to extend life expectancy, and the medicalisation of many aspects of modern life, divorcing people from pain, sickness and death, and becoming unable to cope with life. Illich is regarded as the pioneer of wellness and patient empowerment.

Over the last three decades, wellness and wellbeing has been an area that has grown exponentially, and is reflected in the growth of the 'Natural Health Movement', including complementary therapy, wellness and wellbeing centres and the spa industry. This growth seems characteristic of both developed and emerging markets, with *Express India* (2009) predicting a 30–35 per cent growth in the market for wellness and wellbeing products and services over five years. It is against this backdrop that British politicians became concerned with patients and consumer choice in health and social care. Choice and personalisation was essentially about giving the service user greater control and the ability to choose a setting or a service that corresponded with, and enhanced, their feeling of wellbeing. This is in recognition that health, social care and wellbeing are co-produced, dependent on the engagement, education and involvement of the service user.

In the early years of the new millennium, wellbeing also began to be increasingly used in a variety of areas of social policy, such as mental health and wellbeing (Flateau *et al.*, 2000; Warr, 1990) and children's wellbeing (Camfield *et al.*, 2008). This early dissemination of the term was built around the subjective wellbeing of service users in the policy area concerned. However, objective factors, such as the availability of social and economic resources and the impact of other areas of social policy, including non-functional aspects of vertical social programmes and their silo working, consistently intruded into this discourse. For Camfield *et al.* (2008), 'the objective–subjective distinction is not always helpful, even as a heuristic device, as it obscures the mutually constitutive nature of objective and subjective' (ibid., p. 6).

The separation of administration of social care and health care in much of the UK has long been recognised as problematic for advancing the health and wellbeing of the population. This has led to a variety of policy initiatives to ensure that better care and services are provided and that people's wellbeing is enhanced, including in the following areas.

A statutory duty of partnership

There has been an imperative for partnership working and integration of services to respond to the needs of the individual user, alongside a government-wide commitment to 'joined-up' government at national and local levels. This was reinforced by a statutory duty of partnership between PCTs and NHS Trusts to secure the aims and objectives of the NHS; and also between NHS bodies and local authorities to secure and advance the health and welfare of the people. Legislation for this duty was passed in the Health Act 1999. The government has also issued joint national priorities guidance for the NHS and social services, rather than separate sets of priorities.

Joint Investment Plans

The Joint Investment Plan (JIP) is a key element of the Health Improvement Plan (HImP), designed to improve partnership working between agencies with greater transparency about current and future spending and the development of services at the health/social care interface. The JIP also links with local authority planning arrangements.

New operational flexibilities

Barriers to joint working were replaced by new operational flexibilities, such as:

- Pooled budgets between the NHS and the local authority, with a single accountable officer. However, ultimate accountability links back to existing accountability arrangements for each partner authority.
- Lead commissioning, with one authority able to delegate functions and transfer funding to the other to take responsibility for commissioning both health and social care.
- Integrated provision. While there is no intention to create a situation where the NHS becomes a significant supplier of social care or vice versa, NHS Trusts and PCTs will be allowed to provide some social care services, and social services in-house providers to provide a range of community health services (for example, podiatry and physiotherapy) within the strategies laid down in the HImP and JIP.

Joint inspection and monitoring

There are arrangements for joint inspection and monitoring such as, for example, by the NHS Regional Offices and the Social Care Regional Offices who jointly monitor progress in achieving common objectives and by the Social Services Inspectorate, the Audit Commission and the Care Quality Commission.

Financial incentives

Financial incentives for joint working were seen as one way to stimulate innovation and concentrate effort on specific services. At the same time there was a desire for greater flexibility for authorities to transfer mainstream funds between sectors.

'Wellbeing power'

The full range of collaborative working at local level includes many relevant initiatives of the Blair and Brown administrations (Total Place, LSPs, Local Area Agreements (LAAs) and Multi-Area Agreements (MAAs)). However, the most ambitious attempt to make wellbeing a central focus of policy was the passage of the Local Government Act 2000 (HMSO, 2000). Sections 2 and 5 of Part One set out the details of the 'Wellbeing power'. The way in which this power could be used was detailed in guidance from the DCLG (2009) and the Welsh Office (2009). This power enables eligible councils to do anything that they consider is likely to achieve the promotion or improvement of the economic, social or environmental wellbeing of their area. The government's purpose in this Act was to give communities greater flexibility to act on their priorities and to facilitate joint working between local councils and their partners in the private, public, community and voluntary sectors. This is perceived to provide greater opportunities for local councils to improve the quality of life and health of their communities.

Section 2(1) of the Act enables an eligible council to use the power to promote the economic, social or environmental wellbeing of its area. The wellbeing power provisions are drafted in this way in order to maximise its flexibility. Unless it is specifically restricted by legislation, the power can also be used instead of existing, more specific, powers. For example, where an eligible council has a discretionary power to provide a specific service to a defined group of people, or make a grant to a defined type of organisation, the wellbeing power can be used instead and can also be used to extend the service to other groups or make a grant available to other organisations, where it will improve the wellbeing of individuals, groups or the community as a whole.

Section 2(4) gives councils wide financial latitude, including: the ability to incur expenditure; giving financial assistance to any persons; entering into arrangements or agreements with any person; cooperating with, or facilitating or coordinating the activities of any persons; exercising on behalf of any person any functions of that person; and providing staff, goods, services or accommodation to any person.

Wellbeing in Wales

Guidance from the Welsh Office (2009) extended the DCLG definition of wellbeing to include the achievement of sustainable development. The Welsh guidance gave examples of how the wellbeing powers had been used around the UK. These are illustrated below.

Case study 12.1 Examples of the use of local authority wellbeing powers

Torbay Development Agency

Torbay Council used the wellbeing power to set up a public–private partnership, Torbay Development Agency Ltd, as a company limited by guarantee without share capital. This was a fundamentally new approach, bringing together a variety of functions relating to tourism marketing and development, economic development and regeneration and the management and development of Torbay harbour and its three enclosed harbours.

Social housing in Wakefield

As part of a major regeneration scheme, the power was used to purchase houses on an estate in rapid decline. The use of the power made it possible for the LA to move relatively quickly.

Wood heat technology in Nottinghamshire

Nottinghamshire County Council has been working to develop wood heat technology in schools, installing new boilers or converting existing school boilers to burn wood, to meet its Public Service Agreements (PSA) target to reduce carbon dioxide emissions. The council used the wellbeing power to set up a private non-profit company limited by guarantee, Renewable Utilities Nottinghamshire (RENU) Ltd, to promote the scheme. RENU works to guarantee a quality-assured supply chain for woodchips and wood pellets. It develops relationships with local woodchip suppliers, and undertakes training, awareness raising and fuel screening to ensure quality of supply. The County Council is a minority shareholder in RENU (a 19 per cent stake).

Source: Welsh Office (2009)

CONCLUSION

The previous section painted a picture of the rise of wellbeing, in the UK context, being motivated by disenchantment with modern medicine, a personal quest for wellness and wellbeing, the development of the 'Natural Health Movement', and of considerable commercial interests in wellness and wellbeing. This includes health care professionals cashing in on 'wellness medicine'. Furthermore, the application of notions of wellbeing across many areas of social policy exposed their weaknesses, particularly the way in which silo working and vertical organisations in central and local government worked against the interests of particular service users and communities. This recognition led to a decade of attempts to foster partnership working in LAs and on a regional basis. The unfolding experience of partnership working led to a realisation that control over resources and power to direct and create local policy and matching initiatives also had to be a part of the solution to suboptimal services and suboptimal wellbeing.

The award of wellbeing power to local government in England and Wales has been an organic policy development. However, the impetus for this development lies not only within the UK context described in this chapter. If we look at the wellbeing of the people of the UK in an international and comparative context, the UK performs less well in the published international studies than is suggested by the nationalistic posturing of our politicians and certain professional leaders. For example, the WHO (2000) ranking of national health systems placed the UK as 18th. In respect of the HDI, the UK was ranked 26th (UNDP, 2010). Lowly evaluations on measures of wellbeing have been found in respect of child poverty (UNICEF, 2007), teenage pregnancy rates (Lawlor and Shaw, 2004), income inequality (Duncan, 2000) and educational attainment (PISA, 2010).

Although these studies are not well known among the general public, they provide a backdrop to the 'high politics' of the British state and influence domestic policy. Despite the novelty of the announcement by Prime Minister David Cameron that wellbeing will be measured in the UK, this is old news: DEFRA began to measure wellbeing in 2005, looking both at an overall measure and at various domains of wellbeing suggested by research. The real test for wellbeing is whether explicitly incorporating it into policy making makes governments do different things. The UK Treasury looked at this a few years ago (HM Treasury, 2004), and concluded that the answer was no.

The example from Turkey shows the importance of health security to the wellbeing of a country's citizens. This also mirrors the debates about health care reform in the USA, whose health care system is expensive, inaccessible and performing poorly (Herzlinger, 1997).

Politics, power and policy making are critical elements in the achievement of societal wellbeing. The fact that the achievement of wellbeing requires coordinated and directed action across areas and across programmes means that wellbeing activists need a firm understanding of the policy process, and need to engage in political and policy action if they are to achieve their objectives. The timeliness of this thinking is reflected in the observations of Grace and Whiteman (2010) that 'The Big Society looks to greater citizen responsibility sitting alongside citizens' rights. It envisages more involvement and voluntary effort, and eventually a bigger stock of social cohesion and social glue, (ibid., p.3).

Further reading

House of Commons Communities and Local Government Committee (2009) *The Balance of Power: Central and Local Government Sixth Report of Session 2008–09 Report,* together with formal minutes. London: House of Commons, 12 May

This report looks at the relationship between central and local government in England and argues that it deviates from the European norm in at least three areas: the level of constitutional protection; the level of financial autonomy; and the level of central government intervention. All serve to tilt the balance of power towards the central government.

Froy, F. and Giguère, S. (2008) 'Breaking out of silos: joining up policy locally'

A working paper by the OECD Local Economic and Employment Development Programme. Paris: OECD. This working paper gives a European dimension to the issue of policy and services coordination at local level.

Marks, N. (2005) 'Wellbeing and Social Policy'. Given at Social Policy Association Conference, University of Bath, 29 June. Available at **www.bath.ac.uk/soc-pol/.../spa.../wellbeing-and-public-policy-n-marks.ppt** (accessed 15 August 2011)

This presentation gives an overview of the place of wellbeing in social policy, largely from the viewpoint of subjective wellbeing.

Chapter 13

Public Health, Wellbeing and Culture: A Critical Perspective

Clarence Spigner and Carlos Moreno-Leguizamon

Learning outcome

In this chapter you will learn how to:

- critically discuss the contrasting definition of health and wellbeing in the context of public health discourse;

- critically evaluate the definition of culture as opposed to nation-states, which is an issue in the wellbeing literature.

Modern man believes that he has achieved almost complete mastery over the natural forces which molded his evolution in the past and that he can now control his own biological and cultural destiny. But this may be an illusion. Like all living things, he is part of an immensely complex ecological system and is bound to all of its components by innumerable links. (Dubos, 1959, p. 223)

This chapter problematises the increasing use of the term 'wellbeing' from two perspectives: first, its incremental use at the expense of 'health' without a clear distinction as to what each one means; and second, the crossover of the categories of wellbeing and culture when characterising the level of happiness or life satisfaction of various nation-states, largely from a quantitative perspective.

INTRODUCTION

As the literature shows, wellbeing is used to denote a particular meaning reflective of an individual psychological state of mind, which is indicative of being happy or satisfied with life and its quality. While psychological processes are very much a part of the definition of health, we are concerned about the possible use of the category of wellbeing to convey, arguably, either an integrated conceptualisation of health as a sociocultural, political and economic phenomenon on the one hand or, on the other, a de-socialisation, de-politicisation and de-economisation of the concept of health. In the case of public health, such a uni-dimensional way of constructing the public's health 'muddies the waters', as Cameron *et al.* (2006) state when they note that wellbeing is being used as an open-ended category that comes as a tag attached to health or when health and wellbeing are indistinguishable and the use of both appears somewhat redundant.

Regarding the second issue, which is the crossover of the categories of wellbeing and culture when characterising the level of happiness, life satisfaction or wellbeing of nation-states around the world, this use is confusing in some cases as the literature appears to be portraying nation-states as cultures. This lack of consideration for the range of cultural and other types of human diversity within nation-states amounts to bias and contributes to the perpetuation of stereotypes such as the notion that the people of X or Y country are happier than people from country Z. The aim of this chapter is to suggest that a much more conceptual and methodological clarification is needed in the public health discourse if wellbeing is to be employed as a researchable category from the two perspectives described above.

THE HEALTH OF THE PUBLIC

Foucault (1973) labelled health as having two basic components: the medicine of the species and the medicine of social spaces. The first deals with disease classification, diagnosis, treatment and cure. The second involves disease prevention, intervention and control. Thus, the latter has provided the context in which it is generally accepted that negligent social, economic or political conditions generate unhealthy physical or mental conditions that are largely responsible for disproportionate rates of disease, disability and early deaths in various populations. Morbidity and mortality indicators are determined from a careful analysis of risk factors that occur within populations, and they could come from any angle (for example, genetic, biological, psychological, environmental, social, economic, cultural or political) and not just from the mere notion that individuals are unhappy or dissatisfied with their lives. If the social sciences have played a significant role in contemporary society, it is to bring to the fore the socioeconomic, cultural and political aspects of health that had been relegated to a marginal position by the mainstreaming of health and medical practitioners. Thus, to reduce the use of the category of health by increasing that of wellbeing, without critically thinking about it, could take away gained dimensions that are important in the understanding of public health issues today.

The various general and public health definitions adopted in health policy show how its comprehensiveness as a physical, mental, sociocultural and political event has slowly gained in significance during the last 60 years since the WHO definition in 1948. Again, to exchange this comprehensiveness gained when understanding health issues for an unclear category of wellbeing is risky, particularly when the move from an exclusive biomedical notion of health to a bio-psychosocial one still requires some mainstreaming.

Wolinsky (1988) has pointed to the four basic dualities that haunt modern medicine: 1. reliance on magic and science to cure diseases; 2. an individually oriented and population-based approach to health; 3. consideration for the mind and the body as separate and/or together; and 4. stressing the techno-mechanical rather than the holistic treatment of disease (Wolinsky, 1988, pp. 6–7; also see Carlson, 1975; Moreno-Leguizamon, 2005). It is within this present-day ideologically biased 'biomedical model' perspective that more emphasis tends to be given to the scientific, individually oriented, somatic and technology-driven components of health, along with the positivist 'evidence-based' assessment of contributory etiologies (Riegelman, 2010). Revisiting Wolinsky's dualities, could it be that the increased use of the category of wellbeing, at the expense of the health category in public health, has come to endorse the modern emphasis on the happy or satisfied individual/consumer functioning in a de-politicised, de-socialised and de-economised bubble?

Activity 13.1

The UK government is currently (2010) considering the measurement of wellbeing.

- Suggest at least two characteristics that this measure should cover that would be different from those usually covered in the area of public health.
- How easy was it to come up with the characteristics?

THE DEFINITION OF WELLBEING

The various definitions of wellbeing in the literature reviewed (Bourne, 2010; Cameron *et al.*, 2006; Diener, 2009; NEF, 2004) coincide in addressing the fact that it relates to how individuals evaluate their lives and, in particular, whether they judge them as something desirable, pleasant and good. Describing a brief history of the term, Diener quoting McMahons, summarised it as luck in the Homeric era, virtue in the Aristotelian era, heaven in the Medieval era, pleasure in the Enlightenment era, and probably a 'nice spa' in the contemporary era.

Aristotle's original conceptualisation of wellbeing is fundamental, since it is to him that we owe one of the first characterisations – that of a desirable state of virtue comprising implicitly a norm that encapsulates a judgement about one's life. A second characterisation of the term relates to the judgement that we formulate about our lives in positive terms, namely 'a good life'. This is the one that contemporary economists and psychologists try to quantify, 'scientifically' according to them, using variables such as life satisfaction or quality of life, from a positivist epistemology. The third characteristic relates to the dominance of positive over negative effect, that is, prevalence of pleasant emotions over unpleasant ones. Certainly, the category of wellbeing addresses the experience of the individual, his or her emotions and moods, as well as the assessment of all aspects of his or her life, as suggested by Diener (2009). So, as it is such a subjective category that addresses preferences and choices at the individual level, how does it link to health in general and public health in particular?

The literature reviewed is unclear when defining the relationship between health and wellbeing. McKeown (1979) states that the role of medicine (or health) is not to make people happy but to remove the sources of unhappiness, such as disease and disability (cited in Cockerham, 2007, p. 7). Meanwhile, Barry and Yuill (2008) reiterate how the WHO definition of health was initially 'idealistic and impractical' (Doll, 1992) and that the definition corresponded more to happiness than health (Saracci, 1997). Bourne (2010) considers health to be an indicator of wellbeing. Diener, on the other hand, states that happiness or wellbeing 'leads to better health, better work performance, better social relationships, and to more ethical behavior' (Diener, 2009, p. 66). Cameron *et al.* (2006) consider wellbeing as a component of health. Thus, the various statements show that the relationship between health and wellbeing can be used as interchangeable categories, with one category as the cause (health) and the other one as the effect (wellbeing), or vice versa. It is here that we see the lack of clarity about when to use health and wellbeing as categories in the public health discourse.

When the public health discourse emphasises the role of society/ government as the producer, organiser, regulator and guarantor of the public's health, it seems difficult for it to accommodate the category of wellbeing as a subjective category that addresses preferences and choices at the individual level. So can public health accommodate subjective wellbeing, as defined by Diener, in its discourse? We think it can, if it is clearly understood that public health can lead or contribute to subjective wellbeing and not vice versa. Subjective wellbeing by itself cannot lead or contribute to public health. If the category of subjective wellbeing starts to dominate that of public health, this will probably emphasise the individual aspects over the societal/government aspects. We know that, with the contemporary financial crisis affecting rich and poor governments and societies, there will be greater emphasis on the individual taking care of his or her wellbeing than on the government/ society providing public health. Furthermore, if the individual starts to feel like a consumer of wellbeing rather than health, he or she will probably tend to see it as their duty to pay for it rather than the government/society paying for public health in its role of producer, organiser, regulator and guarantor of the public's health. Obviously, it will be cost-effective for government and societies if wellbeing is promoted at the expense of public health.

If it is accepted that public health contributes to wellbeing, it is also obvious that this wellbeing could take different shapes and forms in terms of ethnicity, gender, class, age, sexual orientation, etc. It is important, for the discourse on public health, to reiterate that behind the subjective experience of the individual and his or her choices concerning subjective wellbeing, there is always society. In the particular case of public health, subjective wellbeing cannot be determinant of the justification of public health discourse.

Similar to the category of wellbeing is 'quality of life', which is defined as 'an individual sense of social, emotional, physical wellbeing which influences the extent in which she or he can achieve personal satisfaction with their life circumstance'. 'Quality of life' usually includes an objective assessment of income, employment and the built environment. But quality of life, similarly to wellbeing, has also emerged with increasing frequency in public health research, teaching and practice. This has led Leidy *et al.* (1999) to report that health-related quality of life (HRQL) is a multidimensional construct encompassing an individual's subjective perceptions of the impact of health status, including disease and treatment, on physical, psychological and social functioning. These broad and multiple uses of wellbeing with quality of life and 'culture' led Kagawa *et al.* (2010) to clarify the relationships between them and to report that quality of life is a 'subjective multi-dimensional experience of wellbeing that is culturally constructed'. This introduces the second issue of interest in this chapter. What is the relationship between wellbeing/life satisfaction and culture?

CULTURE IN PUBLIC HEALTH

In public health discourse, social and cultural dynamics are constructed as shaping population or group-based behaviours, which in turn influence people's emotions and their state of health (Cockerham, 2007; Barry and Yuill, 2008). While related, the state of emotions and state of health can also be mutually exclusive. Meanwhile, culture, as the shared and learnt set of symbols and meanings through which people come to make sense of the world they inhabit, and their behaviours and emotions on a daily basis, allows an integration of the psychological with the cultural. Thus, the cultural context of health comes with the appropriate articulation of etiologies, which are shown to be related to or associated with disability, disease and early death if effective disease prevention, intervention and control are to be a manifestation.

In conducting meaningful public health surveillance, populations and groups are characterised by their cultural contexts and are often epidemiologically categorised by specific circumstances which include time and place. Risk factors or characteristics that increase the probability of suffering disabilities, diseases and early deaths are calculated with the purpose of prevention, intervention and control of those factors (Riegelman, 2010).

Demographics such as race, ethnicity, gender, sexual orientation, age, socioeconomic status or class, occupation, residence, education, political ideology, religion, and regional and/or national affiliation must be clearly designated to prevent, intervene in, and/or control these elements associated with the causes of ill health. Such population-based traits, whether they are ascribed (conferred at birth) or achieved (acquired through individual action), are essential considerations for developing effective public health programmes.

The literature on wellbeing has not so far shown a detailed disaggregation by diverse groups about what it means to them to be happy or satisfied with life. This is particularly true for groups or populations that have been historically marginalised. Far too many studies have chosen entire nation-states to represent a single culture, thereby diminishing the necessary recognition of cultural diversity that exists within so-called 'national' boundaries (Giddens, 1989). The evidence speaks for itself. For instance, Hsiung et al. (2010) studied quality of life among patients with schizophrenia in Taiwan. The concept of culture was broadly defined as 'non-Western'. The self-defined 'subjective quality-of-life indicators' assessed were those of 'mastery, stigma, and social support' among 199 outpatients. Even more expansive about a population defined as a single culture was Terracciano (2005) who, with 87 other colleagues, studied 'national character ratings of 3989 people from 49 cultures'. Kuppens et al. (2008) studied positive and negative emotions regarding 'life satisfaction' among 8557 people from 46 countries. Such self-defined studies about wellbeing with implications for public health have used incredibly large sample sizes, which were not sufficiently articulated to accurately account for the probable 'co-existence of sub-cultures within the society' (Giddens, 1989, p. 737).

In this context, a brief major methodological critical view is needed of what, up to now, seems to have been the major knowledge production of the 'science of wellbeing', as Diener (2009) calls it and reviews it in his detailed book. The methodological approach of the science of wellbeing has so far been mainly quantitative (large statistical surveys) in nature and this has had certain consequences in terms of the assumptions underpinning the research. The problem is not with the statistics themselves but with the strong tendency to generalise from them. Epistemologically, the tendency is based on the premise that research must be objective, without valuation, and almost like the natural sciences. In the 1980s, Johnson and Tuttle, criticising large surveys used to generalise characteristics across societies, stated that:

> inherent in the very notion of sampling are Western assumptions of individual autonomy, egalitarianism, and democracy ... In non-Western cultures, however, the assumptions underlying sampling may be irrelevant. In these cultures where economic circumstances, elites, and authoritarian power structures run counter to sampling's underlying assumptions, the unquestioned use of random sampling will produce a very distorted picture of the society and how it will relate to others. (Johnson and Tuttle, 1989, p. 473)

Along the same lines, another critical observation on large-scale surveys is that correlations simply describe empirical relationships between variables but they do not explain the 'why' of the relationships. Thus, reducing the category of culture to a variable or applying it to the political category of nation-state as equivalent to culture, as has been suggested, is misleading.

Activity 13.2

- What culture or subcultures do you belong to?
- Identify at least three elements that are significant for the wellbeing of your culture or subculture.
- Are these elements particular to your group or common to all in your country?

PUBLIC HEALTH OR A 'SCIENCE OF WELLBEING'?

The public health discourse is multidisciplinary and mainly comprises the biomedical sciences, the social sciences and the humanities. The latter have been playing an increasingly important role (Weed, 1995). However, in the 'science of wellbeing' it has been psychology, with its emphasis on the mental processes of individual human behaviour, that has so far dominated this field of studies. For instance, Diener and Diener (1995) assessed emotional satisfaction among 13 118 college students in 31 nations regarding issues of self-esteem. Other self-defined wellbeing studies about emotions and wellbeing have been conducted by Eid and Diener (2001) and Kuppens et al. (2008). Oishi et al. (2007) studied 'memory and emotion' and Diener et al. (2003) studied 'emotion, personality and culture'. Schimmack et al. (2005) studied 'cultural values' with regard to wellbeing. Diener and Seligman (2002), Lyubomirsky et al. (2005) and Uchida and Kitayama (2009) studied the emotional state of 'happiness' with implications about the state of health. Campbell et al. (2009) also studied 'happiness and social phobia' with implications for health and wellbeing. All these studies were about the subjective state of mind that is indeed part, but certainly not the whole, of health, as this chapter has tried to demonstrate. Bourne's (2010) suggestion that academics should work together and construct an 'operational definition of wellbeing' for better patient care is probably necessary from a more interdisciplinary perspective.

NEF's wellbeing manifesto is significant in the sense that it advocates societal wellbeing, rather than individual wellbeing. NEF's proposal for wellbeing deals with two personal dimensions in combination with one social – the social context: life satisfaction, people's personal development and people's social wellbeing. In relation to the latter, this manifesto argues for some basic social activities, such as how government should really measure what matters, create a wellbeing economy, initiate an education system that promotes flourishing, support a health system that addresses complete health, strengthen civil society and discourage consumerism and gross materialism (NEF, 2004).

In the case of public health, any category of wellbeing with regard to an overall state of health should include evidence-based etiologies (Riegelman, 2010) with direct applications to the social and physical components of human health. As was mentioned earlier, this requirement may be why Cameron *et al.* (2004) strongly cautioned that pushing the concept of wellbeing would only 'muddy the waters' for assessing human health (and especially health policy). Camfield and Skevington (2008) rang similar alarm bells about the too frequently ill-defined use of wellbeing with the concept of health. Thus, as this chapter is trying to demonstrate, a clearer idea of the relationship between public health and wellbeing is needed, along with the use of more qualitative research approaches.

A BRIEF HISTORY OF PUBLIC HEALTH

An historical overview of the public health movement is helpful in clarifying the relationship between health and wellbeing. During the nineteenth century, individualistic attitudes about the health of the public were expressed as 'Social Darwinism' within the 'Spirit of Capitalism' (Hofstader, 1992). Industrial manufacturing forced European peasants off the land into the miserable conditions of factories, while the vile conditions of the transatlantic slave trade of Africans flourished across the colonies (Spigner, 2006–7). Public health casualties occurred as a consequence of the underside of the 'invisible hand'. Edwin Chadwick's *Report on the Sanitation Conditions of the Working Poor in Britain* in 1843, and John Snow's proactive removal of the handle on a public water pump that he deduced to be the common source of London's cholera outbreak of 1854, are among the reformist ideologies of the public health establishment in the UK and the USA (Ham, 2009; Wolinsky, 1988). Undoubtedly, these historical links between the public health movement and the response given by any society, in its capacity as producer, organiser, regulator and guarantor of the public's health, are significant at the moment of understanding the relationship between public health and wellbeing.

Britain's NHS, which was established in 1948, has recently acquired the unflattering label of 'the nanny state', as if the assurance of public access to health was anathematic to self-reliance. In 1976 the Black Report, which was commissioned by the Labour government, showed continuing class inequalities in health (Townsend and Davidson, 1982). By 1998, the release of the Acheson Report, which came after a period of Conservative Party rule, had similar findings and included detailed references to Britain's growing ethnic minority population (Acheson, 1998; Donovan, 1984; Ham, 2009). The age of Thatcher in the UK (1979–90) and Reagan in the USA (1981–9) pushed the free-market principles of health provision inspired by economist Milton Friedman (Friedman and Friedman, 1980). Diseases such as HIV/AIDS, cigarette smoking and rising obesity rates were seen as self-inflicted and were also highlighted in the Wanless Public Health Review (Wanless, 2004).

The 1980s and 1990s were the era of health promotion, during which the individual was targeted for behavioural change (Riegelman, 2010). By 2004, the White Paper *Choosing Health* pointed to an 'approach to support people to make healthy choices in a consumer society' (Ham, 2009, p. 93). Terms such as 'choices' and 'consumer' suggested the individual was somehow now 'free to choose' (Friedman and Friedman, 1980) his or her own health status. Rising health costs helped to shift the political mood, in the UK and USA, towards more individual responsibility for health. In England, publications such as Wilkinson's *Mind the Gap* (2000), Wilkinson and Marmot's *Social Determinants of Health* (2001) and, in the USA, Smedley *et al.*'s *Unequal Treatment: confronting racial and ethnic disparities in health care* (2003) were reminders that more social and fewer individual forces were responsible for increasing inequalities in health. But the notion of personal choice had crept into modern-day health policies. It is against this background that the use of the categories of health and wellbeing need attention.

In the twenty-first century, a more global perspective has emerged in public health, stemming in part from the advent of bio-terrorism, pandemic influenza, global warming and international trading of products ranging from food to toys which have been linked to health problems (Riegelman, 2010). Globalisation has been reflected in many of the wellbeing studies already mentioned (Eid and Diener, 2001; Hsiung *et al.*, 2010; Kuppen *et al.*, 2008; Terracciano, 2005). This proliferation of international research underscores the concern Riegelman has raised that 'population health requires that we define what they mean by a health issue and what we mean by populations' (Riegelman, 2010, pp. 7–8).

BLAME THE VICTIM – BLAME THE CULTURE

As this chapter has attempted to show, specific definitions in health sciences in general, and in public health in particular, are critical since terminology can easily be misinterpreted and misused in social and ultimately political circumstances, with public health implications. For instance, the 'Culture of Poverty' thesis coined by Oscar Lewis (Lewis, 1961) is summarised by Rundall and Wheeler (1979) as an event in which poverty, over time, influences the development of particular social and psychological characteristics among those who are poor. This is essentially a psychological mindset applied to an entire population (in this case, African Americans) with devastating historical, social, political, educational, residential, age-related and racial/ethnic implications (Gans, 1995). The implications are that the poor, the powerless and the marginalised are either blissfully 'happy' with their dismal quality of life or are blamed because of their own self-induced pathology (Auletta, 1982; Leacock, 1971).

Similarly, Nettleton (1995) cited Ahmad (1993) and observed the health effects of intermarriage between second cousins in Britain's Pakistani population. Such endogamous marriages reportedly caused higher levels of autosomal recessive disease (*Lancet*, 1991). But it was also observed that a 'growing number of researchers have begun to hang anything from poor birth outcome to blood disorders, cancers, diseases of the eye and much more onto this new-found explanatory peg' (Nettleton, 1995, p. 187). Such consequences of a specific disease occurring within the 'culture' of Pakistanis in Britain are viewed as both cause and effect because the disease is directly due to the self-imposed lifestyle. Interestingly, the benefits of the 'cousin marriages', independent of the birth outcome, would reflect wellbeing or happiness between the couples.

SELLING AND BUYING WELLBEING

Wellbeing is fast becoming the commercial index of overall health. Riding the wave of free-market enterprise, the category is being used by small businesses as well as large corporations. Wellbeing can be seen in the self-improvement advertisements on the internet. Wellbeing is also the major brand name of a vitamin supplement company in the UK. It is being used to market massage parlours and spas, and to sell relaxation audiotapes and CDs. Wellbeing is used to solicit customers for self-protection services as in 'protect your own wellbeing'. Numerous books now have wellbeing in their titles: books dealing with everything from hedonic psychology to economics to public policy and marriage, children, youth, and the environment. The Wellbeing Institute at the University of Cambridge defines itself as providing 'positive and sustainable characteristics which enable individuals and organizations to thrive'. Local and regional health departments use wellbeing to introduce their departments, programmes, and courses.

CONCLUSION

Wellbeing cannot be the exclusive domain of any ideology, discipline, group, culture, profession, organisation or institution. But the application of the category, as this article demonstrates, has been arbitrary and capricious, especially in the context of the public health discourse (Cameron *et al.*, 2006; Doll, 1992; Saracci, 1997). Also, as this chapter shows, there is the problem of the concept of 'culture' being applied to entire nation-states without considering cultural diversity (Giddens, 1989) within nation-states. Populations or groups, whether defined at the local or the global level, are far too wide-ranging, complex and multidimensional to be so narrowly defined and should therefore be appropriately grouped.

Anthropological and sociological perspectives regarding the concept of culture are generally compatible with public health without blaming the victim. Thus, as Bourne suggests, much work needs to be done to establish some common ground if wellbeing is to be brought more fully into the public health arena.

Further reading

Diener, E. (2009) *The Science of Wellbeing: the collected works of Ed Diener.* New York: Springer Dordrecht

A comprehensive work on wellbeing from a psychological and quantitative perspective.

Bourne, P.A. (2010) 'A conceptual framework of wellbeing in some Western nations'. *Current Research Journal of Social Sciences*, 2(1): 15–23

This article contains a very good definition of wellbeing, although its main discussion comes from an economic perspective.

Cameron, E., Mathers, J. and Parry, J. (2006) 'Health and wellbeing: questioning the use of health concepts in public health policy and practice'. *Critical Public Health*, 16(4): 347–54

An interesting article from the perspective of the relationship between public health and wellbeing.

Chapter 14

Environment and Wellbeing

Veronica Habgood

Learning outcomes

In this chapter you will learn how to:

- contextualise the link between the environment and wellbeing;

- explain the relevance of sustainable development to the maintenance of ecosystems services and their links to human wellbeing;

- consider the environment as both a threat to wellbeing and as an opportunity to promote and enhance wellbeing.

This chapter focuses on wellbeing and the environment. It aims to provide a context for the link between the environment and wellbeing, and considers this link from a conceptual global perspective through a consideration of wellbeing and sustainable development. Through a consideration of environmental quality, the chapter explores how the environment can both promote wellbeing and have an adverse impact on wellbeing, drawing on examples from the UK.

INTRODUCTION: CONTEXTUALISING WELLBEING AND THE ENVIRONMENT

The contribution of the environment to health and wellbeing is acknowledged in the *European Charter on Environment and Health* (WHO, 1989), where 'an environment conducive to the highest attainable level of health and wellbeing' is a stated entitlement. Furthermore, the environment is viewed as a resource that should be managed to improve living conditions and increase wellbeing through a consideration of physical, psychological, social and aesthetic factors. That environmental quality and wellbeing are linked has been acknowledged in a case in the European Court of Human Rights, which accepted that 'severe environmental pollution may affect individuals' wellbeing and prevent them from enjoying their homes in a way as to affect their private and family life adversely, without, however, seriously endangering their health' (Joint Committee on Human Rights, 2008, p. 57). While the links between environmental quality and health are generally well-documented, there is less of an evidence base linking environmental quality and wellbeing. Proposals for a UK wellbeing indicator framework identify 'environment' as a key domain, citing factors such as pollution, countryside and green space, housing and transport (Sustainable Development Commission, 2007).

WELLBEING AND SUSTAINABLE DEVELOPMENT

The UN Millennium Task Force on Environmental Sustainability acknowledges the role that diverse ecosystems play in contributing towards human wellbeing through, for example, the provision of fuel, food and recreational opportunities, but draws attention to the degradation of the environment and the ensuing threats to human wellbeing. This notion of 'ecosystem services' and their role in wellbeing is assessed further by the WHO, which concludes that 'ecosystem services' are indispensable to the health and wellbeing of people everywhere, influencing, for example, good health, social organisation and economic activity (WHO, 2005). Human influence has changed ecosystems to bring about gains in human wellbeing and economic development, but often these changes have an adverse impact on wellbeing. Figure 14.1 presents some of these factors.

Within the context of sustainable development, the need to promote human wellbeing lies at the centre of the need to live within our limits, understand the connections between the economy, society and the environment and ensure equitable distribution of resources and opportunities. It is acknowledged that there are still uncertainties about the linkages between human wellbeing and the provision of ecosystems services generally, although the links with food and water are more clearly understood (WHO, 2005). This uncertainty, however, should not prevent decision makers from taking a precautionary approach to developing policies to safeguard ecosystem services and promote ecologically sustainable development in order to improve health and wellbeing. Such an approach should see not just health but also

Ecosystem service		Examples of human influence on ecosystem services and wellbeing	Constituents of wellbeing
Supporting services Functions necessary for all ecosystem services: • nutrient cycling; • water cycling; • soil formation; • primary production.	**Provisioning services** Products we obtain from ecosystems: • food; • fresh water; • wood and fibre; • fuel.	• Increasing demand for food. • Overfishing and exploitation of wild food. • Deforestation. • Inadequate sanitation and access to clean water. • Depletion of fossil fuels.	**Basic material for good life:** • shelter; • sufficient nutritious food; • adequate livelihoods; • access to goods.
	Regulating services Benefits we obtain from the regulation of ecosystem services: • climate regulation; • flood regulation; • disease regulation; • water purification.	• Air pollution from combustion of fossil and biomass fuels. • Uncontrolled management of waste. • Irrigation and damming. • Loss of biodiversity.	**Security:** • personal safety; • secure access to resources; • security from disasters.
Cultural services Non-material benefits derived from ecosystem services: • aesthetic experience; • spiritual enrichment; • educational; • recreation/tourism.		• Population migration. • Urbanisation and uncontrolled development. • Technological innovation. • Transportation systems. • Economic and political instability. • Conflict.	**Health:** • feeling well; • access to clean air and water; • strength. **Good social relations:** • social cohesion; • mutual respect; • ability to help others.

Figure 14.1 Ecosystem Services, the Constituents of Wellbeing and Human Influence (adapted from WHO 2005 and UK National Ecosystem Assessment 2010)

wellbeing as a consideration when preparing national or local policy and regulatory impact assessments. For example, guidance has been provided by the UK Department of Health to support those preparing a health and wellbeing statement for a Regulatory Impact Assessment (DH, 2009). More examples of this type of guidance are anticipated as the UK develops an ecosystems approach to policy and decision making.

Activity 14.1 An ecosystems approach to wellbeing

While the world's poorest populations depend disproportionately on ecosystem services for their wellbeing, richer countries are also reliant on what the environment can offer to promote wellbeing. For example, in the UK since 1945 the conversion of semi-natural habitats to arable land, coupled with the greater intensity in agricultural production and use of agro-chemicals, has resulted in gains in terms of food production but a loss in biodiversity and the degradation of, for example, aquatic environments (UK National Ecosystem Assessment, 2010). In another example, 90 per cent of the UK population lives in urban areas where high-density housing, the sale of playing fields and lack of funding for public parks can limit the availability of green space (UK National Ecosystem Assessment, 2010).

Can you think of other examples of human influence on ecosystems services and wellbeing in the UK?

WELLBEING AND ENVIRONMENTAL QUALITY

Environmental quality may be defined as the 'properties and characteristics of the environment, that impact on human beings and other organisms' (European Environment Agency, 2010). Characteristics may include the extent to which air or water are polluted, the presence of noise, access to green space, the visual effects of buildings and urban design (European Environment Agency, 2010).

A body of evidence that identifies wellbeing as a function of ambient environmental quality is now beginning to emerge. Studies by Rehdanz and Maddison (2006) on local environmental quality and life satisfaction in Germany conclude that subjective wellbeing is diminished by perceptions of poor local air quality and high levels of noise. Another study focusing on the environment and mental wellbeing, undertaken in Greenwich, London, found that the two most important environmental factors influencing mental wellbeing were access to green space and neighbour noise (Guite *et al.*, 2006). A study of life satisfaction and ambient air quality in London found a strong negative association between life satisfaction and both perceived and measured poor air quality in respect of the pollutant nitrogen dioxide (NO_2), and concluded that the findings lend further credibility to the arguments for improving air quality which, to date, have focused on improving public health, meeting a legal imperative and achieving climate change reduction (MacKerron and Mourato, 2009). The next part of this section looks at some of these aspects of environmental quality.

Urban design and wellbeing

Pacione (2003) discusses the concept of the 'liveable city', in which consideration is given to meeting the social, economic and environmental needs of the population. The condition of the environment in which people live and work can influence their wellbeing. Crime, litter, graffiti and other forms of vandalism degrade the liveability of the environment and reduce the perception of safety. This perception of local nuisance and safety influences the extent to which people engage in physical activity and rate their health status (Sustainable Development Commission, 2008).

Strong communities, social cohesion and physical activity that enables people to live healthy, fulfilling lives can be promoted by attention to the design and maintenance of rural and urban environments (Sustainable Development Commission, 2008). CABE (2009) propose that planners should work with health professionals to integrate health and wellbeing into approaches that guide development. Some of the key approaches that are proposed by CABE to promote wellbeing through good urban design include:

- integrating the design of green space into both new-build and regeneration projects;
- planning development that discourages road traffic and promotes sustainable transport, including pedestrian and cycling routes;
- providing local services as a focal point of neighbourhoods;
- designing and maintaining places that look cared for, discourage vandalism and enhance the perception of safety.

Green space and wellbeing

It has been suggested that there is a connection between sustainable public health and sustainable natural environment agendas (Stone, 2006), and there has been growing interest in initiatives promoting access to green space as a means to improve health and wellbeing. The Royal Commission on Environmental Pollution (2007) advocates that access to green space can promote good health, wellbeing and quality of life. One of the most commonly cited benefits is improvement in mental wellbeing but, clearly, access to green space can promote greater physical activity with the concomitant benefits of improved health. The benefits to wellbeing as a consequence of access to green space are evident in all sections of society (Natural England, 2008):

- improvements in children's social, mental and physical development;
- improvements in concentration and self-discipline for children exhibiting symptoms of ADHD;
- the promotion of healthy ageing;
- a contribution towards more cohesive communities with a sense of identity and less crime;
- facilitates adults to live more productive, active and fulfilling lives.

Newton (2007) provides a broad definition of 'green space' as including woodlands and forest, agricultural land, rural landscapes, nature reserves and parks and urban green spaces (for example, gardens, parks, allotments and tree-lined walkways). The contribution of green space to improvements in wellbeing and health is beginning to develop a strong evidence base. For example, O'Brien (2006) cites a number of studies that focus on the extent to which trees, woodland and green spaces contribute towards physical, psychological and social wellbeing. Benefits accrue, not just from being physically active within green spaces, but also from being in close proximity to them.

However, the notion of 'ecotherapy' is not a new idea. Mind (2007) cites the green and leafy surroundings of the mental health institutions of the past by way of example, but expresses concern that 'ecotherapy' is not widely regarded as a serious treatment option for those with a mental health illness.

A number of initiatives focusing on encouraging the use of woodland have been funded in the UK. While not specifically focusing on wellbeing outcomes, a Forestry Commission project (O'Brien and Morris, 2009) involving five woodland sites in England reported the benefits of access to woodland as:

- socialising;
- contact with nature;
- mental and physical health improvements;
- a sense of achievement and self-improvement;
- enjoyment;
- positive influences on other areas of life and improvements in general wellbeing.

The extent to which people access green space has been shown to be associated with their proximity. In the USA it was found that those people living within one mile of a park were four times more likely to visit the park than those living further away (Cohen *et al.*, 2007). It is suggested that the beneficial effects of green space on health and wellbeing are not routinely considered by policy makers, particularly in relation to spatial planning in urban areas, and concerns are expressed about the impact on lower socioeconomic groups where the pressures on urbanisation put pressure on urban green space (Groenewegen *et al.*, 2006). Natural England (2010) proposes, in its green space standards, that every house should be within 300 m of an area of green space of at least 2 ha and, in order to promote this, has signed a concordat with the UK Public Health Association, NHS Alliance and the Faculty of Public Health that supports the concept of the 'Natural Health Service'.

The Natural Health Service

The overarching aim of the Natural Health Service is to bring about improvements in health and wellbeing through access to green space, working through local strategic partnerships, local area agreements and the third sector:

> We believe that everyone should have the right of access to local, high quality, natural green space to benefit their physical and mental health and wellbeing. (Natural England, 2009)

Our Natural Health Service is linked to the Change4Life initiative ('Eat well, move more, live longer') and aims to:

1. Increase the number of households within a five-minute walk of an area of green space of at least 2 ha.
2. Enable every GP or community nurse to be able to signpost patients to an approved health walk or outdoor activity programme.

> The Faculty of Public Health calls for a partnership approach involving policy makers, town planners, public health practitioners, health professionals, the voluntary sector, community groups, local media and the public to harness the potential use of green space for health and wellbeing (Faculty of Public Health, 2010).

Research by Natural England (2010) reveals that 54 per cent of the adult population in England visit the natural environment each week, although 10 per cent had not visited in the previous 12 months and a further 8 per cent had made just one or two visits. Visits to the natural environment appear more prevalent in those aged 45–64, those in employment and those in the higher socioeconomic groups (Natural England, 2010). Those with a disability and black and minority ethnic groups are less likely to use green space (Croucher *et al.*, 2008). The 'Outdoors for All' action plan aims to reconnect under-represented groups with the natural environment and supports the provision of green space for those affected by health inequalities (DEFRA, 2008).

Although green space may not be accessed specifically for physical exercise, participation in green exercise activities offers benefits to health and wellbeing. The Green Gym® ('Green Gym' is a registered trademark of the British Trust for Conservation Volunteers) is a programme overseen by the British Trust for Conservation Volunteers (BTCV) that aims to provide people with a way to enhance their fitness and health while taking action to improve the outdoor environment. While not specifically focusing on improving wellbeing, this, clearly, is an additional outcome. The BTCV also coordinates a 'Wellbeing Comes Naturally' initiative, which aims to improve people's mental and physical health through environmental activity and, especially, targets those with mental distress.

Case Study 14.1 The Green Gym® in Camden, London

The BTCV Green Gym® is a scheme that inspires individuals to improve both their health and wellbeing and the environment at the same time. Through programmes such the Green Gym® and promotion of a 'natural health service', BTCV will provide opportunities for 500 000 people to become fitter and improve their mental health between 2009 and 2013 (BTCV, 2009). The Green Gym® in Camden is one such scheme, run in partnership with the London Borough of Camden, NHS Camden, Royal Parks and Mind.

The aim of the scheme, which is free to all adults, is to 'combine physical activity with the feel-good factors of working with a team, learning new skills, improving the environment and being outdoors' (BTCV, 2010). The group meets at various green space locations such as parks and nature reserves within the London Borough of Camden. Each session begins with a 'warm up', includes light refreshments and concludes with a 'cool down'.

Work within Camden includes: planting orchards, bulbs and native hedgerows; improving habitats for insects and other wildlife; supporting and establishing community food-growing projects; clearing invasive plants to maintain rare habitats; litter clearance, coppicing and improving access to community green space. Some of the activities contribute towards Mind's 'Time to Change' programme.

The Green Gym® scheme was recognised by the *Guardian* newspaper as one of the ten best free things to do in the summer of 2010.

Activity 14.2 Access to green space

Think about the locality in which you live. What opportunities are there for access to green space? To what extent is this green space available to all members of the community? What improvements could be made to enhance the wellbeing and health benefits of the green space that is available?

Blue space and wellbeing

More recently, the concept of 'blue space' has emerged, promoting the use of coastal and other aquatic environments to enhance health and wellbeing. Depledge and Bird (2009) draw attention to the Victorian practice of convalescence in seaside locations, and it was common practice in the northern industrial towns of England for there to be day trips to the nearest coastal resort.

Evidence from Australia suggests that those living closer to coastal areas are more likely to be physically active (Bauman *et al.* 1999, cited in Depledge and Bird, 2009), and Depledge and Bird (2009, p. 948) argue that 'the presence of the sea motivates outdoor activity and enhances wellbeing', but there is little evidence specifically referring to blue space and wellbeing. A new initiative, the Blue Gym, based on the success of the Green Gym®, discussed above, has been launched to gather evidence on the extent to which health and wellbeing benefits arise from access to coastal environments.

Case Study 14.1 The 'Blue Gym'

The UK is well placed to promote access to coastal environments to improve health and wellbeing, with nowhere being further than 73 miles from the coast. It is considered that the coast and inland waterways of the UK have untapped potential to yield health and wellbeing benefits, and the Peninsula Medical School in Plymouth, supported by the Environment Agency, Natural England and the Department of Health, aims to create a national network of Blue Gym activities that specifically promote the mental and physical health benefits of participation in exercise along the coast and in other aquatic environments.

Research is being conducted to explore the extent to which water-based activities are associated with the following benefits:

- increased physical activity;
- improvements in mental health and wellbeing;
- a greater understanding of inland waterways and coastal environments;
- improvements to the natural environment from conservation activity.

The benefits to physical and mental wellbeing will be assessed by asking participants to complete a 'Water and Wellbeing' questionnaire. Examples of projects include:

- 'Walking the Coastal Way to Health' – guided walks to enable those with physical and mental health issues to spend more time around aquatic environments (in conjunction with the National Marine Aquarium);

- 'Share the Smile' – designed to pair up watersports enthusiasts with novices to enable them to experience watersports (in conjunction with the Environment Agency);
- 'Surf for Success' – a surf-based activity for children with emotional and behavioural issues (in conjunction with Globalboarders Ltd);
- 'Tectona' – a sail-training organisation for young people and those with various mental health issues.

Noise and wellbeing

Noise is commonly defined as 'sound which is undesired by the recipient' (Wilson Committee, 1963). While sound can damage hearing, the human response to noise is subjective and might depend on the nature, intensity and duration of the noise; its frequency and time of occurrence; what individuals are doing; individual sensitivity; and the extent of any economic links with the source of the noise.

Noise, from whatever source, can have an impact on health and wellbeing; indeed, the manner by which noise in a community is often judged actionable is determined not by its potential direct impact on health, but whether or not it constitutes a 'nuisance'. While full discussion of 'nuisance' is precluded in this publication, it has at its core considerations for an individual's wellbeing and enjoyment of their land.

Road traffic noise is often identified as the most dominant source of noise in urban environments, but it is not the most common source of complaint to local authorities in the UK. Local authorities receive most complaints about noise from domestic premises ('neighbour noise') (Chartered Institute of Environmental Health, 2010). The effects of environmental noise on health and, to a lesser extent, wellbeing, particularly in urban environments, have been examined most especially in connection with the impacts of traffic and aircraft noise. Speech communication activities, such as watching television, are those most disturbed by aircraft noise, whereas sleep disturbance is more significant for traffic noise (Stansfeld and Matheson, 2003). Exposure to road traffic noise can result in sleep disturbance and non-auditory impacts such as increased fatigue, decreased wellbeing, annoyance, behavioural changes and deterioration in performance (Bluhm *et al.*, 2004).

Annoyance is a function of perceived noise and may manifest itself as 'fear' or 'mild anger', and appears to be related to the extent to which noise interferes with everyday activities (Stansfeld and Matheson, 2003). Annoyance generally increases with noise exposure and, while a degree of habituation to environmental noise is not uncommon, the periodicity of road traffic and aircraft noise events (such as the passing of an HGV) may be such that habituation occurs to a lesser extent than, for example, exposure to industrial noise. Annoyance may not result in serious physical health effects, but has been shown to have a negative effect on quality of life and psychological wellbeing.

Gidlöf-Gunnarsson and Öhrström (2007) conclude that psychological wellbeing can be improved by reducing exposure to noise, and call for greater access to green space to mitigate the effects of noise, a reduction in road traffic noise and the need to design 'noise free' indoor and outdoor space. In the UK, local authorities are well equipped with legislative tools to deal with neighbour noise, but the approach to road traffic and aircraft noise must be proactive and planned. European legislation already prescribes maximum sound levels for motor vehicles and motorcycles, so it is incumbent upon local authorities to use planning policy and legislation to mitigate the potential impact of road traffic noise on wellbeing. Noise action plans provide a framework for managing environmental noise in the most noisy agglomerations, particularly from traffic, railways and aircraft, and aim to preserve quiet areas (DEFRA, 2010b). Some local authorities are beginning to develop noise strategies.

Case study 14.2 City of Westminster Noise Strategy

The major source of noise in the City of Westminster is road traffic, and 37 per cent of residents questioned said that road traffic noise had bothered them in the last 12 months (City of Westminster, 2010). Average daytime and night-time noise levels in Westminster exceed the WHO guidelines for community noise.

The City of Westminster has introduced a noise strategy for the period 2010–15, the main aim being to contribute towards improving the health and wellbeing of residents, workers and visitors. The strategy has four key objectives (City of Westminster, 2010):

- reduce noise levels;
- reduce noise incidents;

- minimise the impact of noise on noise-sensitive development;
- protect and create tranquil areas and sounds with positive associations.

The strategy presents short-, medium- and long-term actions. Examples of proposed actions to reduce road traffic noise include:

- promoting quieter modes of transport such as walking, cycling and the use of electric vehicles;
- noise-reduction schemes along roads under Westminster's control;
- using quieter road surfacing materials;
- restrictions, where possible, on the types of vehicle using certain roads, for example, coaches and HGVs.

CONCLUSION

The environment clearly plays a role in the maintenance, promotion and enhancement of human wellbeing, and the evidence base is growing. This chapter has shown how changes to, and degradation of, ecosystems services can bring about both improvements and disbenefits to wellbeing. The principles of sustainable development provide a context and rationale for policy and action at a global and local level to ensure that wellbeing, as well as health, is prioritised and promoted. Wellbeing, however, is a multidimensional state and further research is needed to explore the relationship between the environment and both objective and subjective elements of wellbeing.

In the UK, the benefits to wellbeing of the environment are now being recognised and a range of national and local initiatives is evident, largely focusing on the natural environment. A partnership approach is needed to identify and further develop the opportunities presented by both natural and man-made environments. Joined-up thinking across a range of disciplines during the development of policy will maximise the synergies between the environment and wellbeing.

Further reading and useful websites

Mind: Time to Change.
Available at www.time-to-change.org.uk/about-us

This is a programme that aims to end discrimination faced by people who experience mental health problems and includes projects, activities and events that promote wellbeing.

SHEBEEN. Available at http://s207555923.websitehome.co.uk

The aim of SHEBEEN is to promote the greater social inclusion and empowerment of Sheffield's black and ethnic minorities in relation to the built, human and natural environment.

BTCV Green Gym. Available at www2.btcv.org.uk/display/greengym

The Blue Gym.
Available at www.bluegym.org.uk/page/about-blue-gym-1
Contact: Dr Mat White, University of Plymouth.

Acknowledgements

Chris Speirs, BTCV Green Gym, Camden for permission to use the Green Gym at Camden as a case study.

Dr Mat White, University of Plymouth for permission to use the Blue Gym as a case study.

Chapter 15

Housing, the Built Environment and Wellbeing

Jill Stewart and Fiona Bushell

Learning outcomes

In this chapter you will learn how to:

- differentiate between housing and health and housing and wellbeing, understanding the fundamental role of housing and communities in the overall wellbeing of society;

- evaluate the contribution of the design of the built environment to wellbeing;

- understand the importance of housing and social care in maintaining and promoting positive mental (emotional) health and wellbeing through the lifespan;

- discuss the potential of collaborative working in promoting wellbeing, such as through Joint Strategic Needs Assessments.

This chapter explores the interplay between housing, health and wellbeing. For the purposes of this chapter, wellbeing in housing and the built environment is about individuals and communities enjoying a healthy home and living environment, enhanced through active participation and citizenship, quality and enjoyment of life with physical, social, economic and psychological needs being met. This chapter demonstrates that wellbeing is enhanced by decent, secure and affordable housing and a good built environment throughout the lifespan, meeting appropriate needs from early childhood and into older age.

INTRODUCTION

Although wellbeing may be a relatively new policy term, it is far from a new concept in terms of housing and built environment developments. As far back as the 1890s, Ebenezer Howard's Garden City movement recognised some of the challenges of overcrowded and poor urban living environments and the need for better housing within greener living environments. Overall this fostered a new approach to physical, cultural, environmental and social planning ideals before the full-scale development of local councils providing and managing social housing after the First World War. While many housing developments provided good-quality housing and environments, some high-rise tower block estates designed and developed from the 1950s failed to become the modern living utopia initially envisaged, and some are now associated with low levels of wellbeing (for further reading, see 'Health, Safety and Wellbeing in Housing' chapter in Rhoden, forthcoming).

In the run-up to the 2010 General Election, the Chartered Institute of Housing launched its HouseProud campaign. The campaign's objectives were to raise the profile of the fundamental importance of housing and support services in society, since they lie at the heart of promoting health, and social and economic wellbeing, and to help ensure a dynamic national and strategic approach for housing.

THE DESIGN OF THE BUILT ENVIRONMENT AND WELLBEING

Recent policy on sustainable communities and neighbourhood renewal has used a place-centred approach (DCLG, 2009) (see Box 15.1). Place matters because the environment can either support or limit physical, mental, emotional, spiritual and social health and wellbeing (DCLG, 2009; Cavill, 2007; Guite et al., 2006; ODPM, 2005a; Williams and Green, 2001). The design of places has an impact on the environment, people and sustainable development (CABE, 2009; DH 2009; ODPM, 2005; Williams and Green, 2001). Guite et al. (2006) confirmed an association between the physical environment and mental wellbeing across a range of domains, the most important factors being neighbourhood noise, a sense of overcrowding in the home and escape facilities such as green spaces and community facilities, and fear of crime. Thus, Guite et al. (2006) suggest there is a need for careful consideration of design and social features of residential areas to promote mental wellbeing. Their study also confirmed that liking the look of where you live is important to mental health.

Halpern (1995, cited in Guite *et al.*, 2006) highlighted the importance of the involvement of residents in the planning process, in particular with regard to aesthetics, as there is often a difference between the public's view of good building design and the views of the architects. Despite government guidance, Cavill (2007, p. 18) suggests that 'it is still uncommon for new building at any significant scale to reflect the national agenda promoting pedestrian-friendly, human-orientated development, which can help to strengthen and foster community'.

Box 15.1 Sustainable communities policies

- The National Strategy for Neighbourhood Renewal (Social Exclusion Unit, 2001), a place-based approach whereby no one should be seriously disadvantaged by where they live, aims to reduce inequalities by regenerating the most deprived areas and giving local communities greater ownership.
- *Sustainable Communities: people, places and prosperity* (ODPM, 2005) – a focus on place – the government's five-year plan aimed at giving local residents more influence and power to improve their lives and more say over what happens where they live. Sustainable communities are defined as places where people want to live and work now and in the future, that meet the needs of existing and future residents, are sensitive to their environment and contribute to a high quality of life. They are safe, inclusive, well planned, built and run and offer equality of opportunity and good services for all. For communities to be sustainable they must offer decent affordable homes, good public transport, schools, hospitals, shops, a clean safe environment and open public space where people can relax and interact, and an ability to have a say on the way their neighbourhood is run.
- *Strong and Prosperous Communities: the local government white paper* (DCLG, 2006), a focus on neighbourhoods, partnership and participation. It reflects the principles of a place-focused approach by aiming to improve the relationship between different vertical and horizontal levels of decision making and cross-sector working. It includes bringing together in LSPs responsibilities for preparing a Sustainable Community Strategy, the Local Development Framework and LAA. Community Strategies put a strong, sustainable and cohesive community at the heart of their vision and part of this is individual wellbeing and development, a safe, secure and attractive environment

---

together with economic opportunity and prosperity.

- *Place Matters* (DCLG, 2007), a vision of 'prosperous and cohesive communities, offering a safe, healthy and sustainable environment for all' and putting 'place' at the heart of what it does.
- *World Class Places: the government's strategy for improving quality of place* (DCLG, 2009), aiming to improve how places are planned, designed, developed and maintained.

Better buildings and spaces improve quality of life and make places safer and, together with a strong identity and local character, make people feel valued and encourage pride and sense of place (CABE, 2009). Successful design fosters health-promoting environments (Arts Council England, 2005). Design and space management affect how the buildings are used and can aid way finding. 'Siting, landscaping, creative use of materials, colour and works of art help to communicate a sense of personalised care, rather than an institutional service' (CABE, 2009, p. 15). Healthy, therapeutic places are welcoming, accessible, relaxing and comfortable. They put people in control of their environment and in contact with the natural environment, exploit natural light, use natural ventilation and are designed to reduce energy use (CABE, 2009).

Design turns architecture into a relationship with the user but requires imagination, collaboration and a reduction in bureaucratic barriers. Creative, beautiful design using an exciting layout, colour, light, innovative shapes and materials can lift the spirits, affect mood and emotions, increase service-user numbers, boost productivity, improve pupil achievement, change behaviour and enhance social relationships (DCLG, 2009; Arts Council England, 2005).

Ecological considerations need to be integrated into approaches to health and wellbeing (Nurse *et al.*, 2010). City landscaping involving plants can reduce urban heat and encourage wildlife. Materials should be used that reduce carbon emissions and are sustainable. There should be a green infrastructure with sustainable transport networks to enable healthy lifestyles, as access to quality green space promotes mental health, relieves stress, overcomes isolation, improves social cohesion and alleviates physical problems (CABE, 2009).

REGENERATION AND WELLBEING

Regeneration schemes have been shown to have a positive effect on the health and wellbeing of residents (Williams and Green, 2001). A Channel 4 series (McCloud, 2008) in Castleford, Yorkshire demonstrated the issues that need to be addressed for successful regeneration. The regeneration initiative lasted over five years, between 2003 and 2008. It started with £100 000 of Channel 4 money invested in the regeneration of this former mining town and residents have since raised £6 million through two regeneration agencies, the Arts Council and local council. See Table 15.1.

What worked?	Barriers	Sense of place
• Derelict wasteland became parks.	• Long delays, bureaucracy.	• New energy and hope for the future.
• Architect listened.	• Architect not listening to residents.	• Families intend to stay.
• Architect researched history of area.	• Tight budget.	• Attitudes changed as buildings and streets changed.
• Security measures.	• Cutting-edge architecture – too much change.	• Safer place.
• Relocation of market to centre.	• Lack of belief/vision in architect.	• Empowerment of residents.
• Elegant new bridge.	• Too much of a compromise.	• School parliament.
• Transformation of streets.	• Facilities not robust enough.	• Sense of ownership/ambition.
• Traffic calming.	• Mismatch of designers and community and poor communication.	• Beautiful design and pride.
• Entrance to town inviting.		
• Community champions.	• Mis-spending of money on works other agencies can do.	• Community spirit.
• Tenacity, commitment and energy.	• Change in responsibility for funding.	• Attracting business/investment.
• Funding agencies giving residents control.	• Sponsors dictating projects – not always creative.	• Sustainability – projects maintained by community and have led to others.
• Collaboration, partnership, consultation.	• Lack of community champion for all projects.	
• Investment – shops, library, museum, business centre.		

Table 15.1: What makes successful regeneration schemes?

Box 15.2 Examples of design that enhances wellbeing

Idea Store (2006)

Whitechapel Market, East End of London, was a public library, not used much so it was rebranded. The London Borough of Tower Hamlets provided a modern interior influenced by urban style. The Idea Store offers adult education classes, dancing, music and drama. Libraries have to be relevant to people. Visual language – green and blue stripes is a common motif of market canopies. No foyer – opens out to the street at ground level. Sitting people at windows keeps them in contact with landscape. Modern, sparkling and bright. Increased visitor numbers reflecting ethnic mix, more accessible to all.

Westminster Academy School (CABE, 2010)

Dense urban environment sandwiched between commuter route and M40 flyover. An example of an underachieving school in a deprived area turned around through quality, simple, modern, imaginative design. Colour, motivational words, neon lights, sports hall used by community, huge atrium. Children feel safe, secure, CCTV, swipe cards, anti-bullying toilets. Children want to learn and feel valued. Scattered breaks, acoustic separation. Building changes behaviour – has effect on lives.

Villiers High School in Southall (Design Council, 2009)

Designing out crime. Teenagers of 35 different nationalities had to use an empty tarmac space each lunchtime and fights broke out. Students pitched to Ealing council for £25 000 to fund a collaborative design and build project. The regenerated space gives students space but allows staff to see what's happening and stop conflicts. The students wanted to do something about the violence and were involved from the start. The designer observed how the students used the space and why. Colourful concrete blocks give students their own spaces, lots of open space, and encourage ownership and pride. A climbing wall encourages activity. Now more students use the space and there is no violence.

Staiths South Bank Gateshead (CABE, 2010)

A collaboration between property developers and the community in the development of affordable houses. Space for kids to grow and play. Places designed for people, not profit. Largest new build Home Zone, creative landscaping and social spaces to encourage interaction.

Beddington Zero Energy Development (BedZED) (Bioregional, 2010)

The UK's largest mixed-use sustainable community. A variety of one-bedroom apartments to four-bedroom houses to own or rent, all with outside space that can be personalised. A green lifestyle with sky gardens, wind cowls, super-insulated buildings, and local food-growing and car clubs. Careful design with public space for meetings, child friendly, no cars in centre. Higher quality of life. Green roofs help alleviate environmental damage. Reduce urban heat/increase biodiversity. Can have roofs at people level, parks on top of car parks. Put back soil and vegetation – good for soul and wellbeing.

THE COMMUNITY AND WELLBEING

As we have seen, housing and wellbeing is not just about bricks and mortar. There has been increasing recognition of the ways in which neighbourhood conditions can affect health, and that community cohesion and community participation can have positive effects on health. Social capital is the 'glue' holding society together and this can help promote a sense of belonging, trust, support and capacity, and is therefore a positive community resource and attribute (Swann and Morgan, 2002), which is recognised as important in strengthening marginal communities and reducing health inequalities.

Many deprived areas are very deficient in social capital and those living in such areas are more likely to suffer stress through loneliness, isolation and fear of crime. Such a breakdown in social fabric can be enormously challenging to address. Sensitive local facilities and services are required to encourage more active citizenship, and younger children in particular may be more open and tolerant to change, which may have important implications for their longer-term wellbeing (Cattrell and Herring, 2002). Generally speaking, communities rich in social capital are also socially cohesive and active as local people work together, gaining mutual and supportive benefit. Such a neighbourhood or community can help provide a basis for community development and this is fundamental in supporting sustainable physical regeneration strategies, although active local people may become easily demotivated by bad experiences (Cattrell and Herring, 2002).

Regeneration strategies need to involve local communities if they are to be successful and sustainable, and successful in promoting wellbeing. Many residents of more deprived areas may already suffer 'regeneration fatigue' and the history should be taken into account when planning sensitive regeneration initiatives, dealing with each area in a unique and appropriate culturally sensitive way. Engagement and community cohesion are important in regeneration. Dealing with diverse and 'hard to reach' communities can be particularly challenging, requiring skilled strategies and interventions to be successful and sustainable. Capacity building is also important to nurture and train local people in strengthening the community's skills, abilities and confidence to gain a greater sense of power over their lives (Lister *et al.*, 2007).

HOUSING AND WELLBEING THROUGH THE LIFESPAN

Decent housing provides a cornerstone throughout the lifespan for wellbeing and quality of life and, as such, it follows that good housing in a good environment from 'the cradle to the grave' is fundamental to the wellbeing agenda. Prioritising children is important in addressing inequality (Wilkinson and Marmot, 2003), with physical and mental health benefits (Marmot *et al.*, 2010). Children born into decent housing are more likely to enjoy and maintain positive mental health, including quality social interaction from the outset, while those born, for example, into temporary accommodation or low-quality marginal social housing are less likely to benefit.

Poor housing can lead to poor mental or emotional health for a range of reasons. For example, already deprived households may only be able to access the bottom end of the privately rented sector, such as houses in multiple occupation, suffering poor-quality housing and the constant threat of eviction. Children in temporary and/or overcrowded accommodation have a higher risk of being exposed to other residents with mental health, drug and alcohol problems, and risk missing out on regular health care or education. Poor-quality, polarised social housing estates may suffer low levels of social capital and capacity. Communities or individuals may fear crime or suffer stress through noise nuisance. Older people may be isolated and lonely in their homes, and at higher risk of home accident. Lower income groups may suffer fuel poverty due to high fuel prices and poor-quality housing and heating appliances (for further discussion, see Stewart *et al.*, 2005).

An ageing population

With a rapidly ageing population, housing and allied social care services need to be able to respond appropriately and sensitively to promote wellbeing for older people. Older people are the most likely to occupy non-decent homes and require social care services, and there is a need for a greater understanding of housing and health links as well as the housing and social care interventions available to help independent living and chronic health condition management (Adams, 2007; Donald, 2009). There is a growing body of literature demonstrating the importance of people being able to remain independently in their own homes, supported by appropriately tailored social and care services (see, for example, Croucher *et al.*, 2006). Particular attention needs to be given to lower income households in the private housing sector (both owner occupiers and tenants), where residents risk missing out on services, even though they may comprise a particularly isolated community where well-considered and targeted interventions can be highly effective in quality of life and independence, although front-line staff need to be appropriately trained and resourced (Allan, 2005).

As the population ages, there are intense challenges facing the housing and wellbeing agenda, and poverty, isolation and growing frailty will become increasingly important factors facing policy makers. Age Concern (2008) demonstrates the challenges for older people in meeting housing and social care costs which are crucial to independence, health and wellbeing. The number of people with progressive conditions such as dementia will also increase (Habell, 2010), which will bring housing and social care needs to the fore across all housing tenures. Many in the private housing sector may be isolated and vulnerable, particularly those living alone or those whose carers are struggling to assist as their own condition deteriorates.

As the number of those with dementia rises, social landlords are likely to play an important role as residential schemes require extra care provision, while maintaining as much independence as possible. Purpose-designed housing can help provide appropriate accommodation and allow for a carer to remain with their partner. More successful schemes have had necessary features 'designed in' to help provide the best accommodation possible to enhance wellbeing. Design features include:

- good lighting and ventilation;
- adequately sized rooms for proper circulation (residents, visitors, staff, familiar furniture);
- low windows to enable bed-ridden or chair-bound residents to see out;
- level surfaces (including access to lifts, etc.);
- gas monitors to cut off the gas supply if it has been left on;
- door sensors to alert help where appropriate;
- colour coding and personalisation to help residents recognise their accommodation;
- glass-fronted kitchen units to help visual recognition;
- a single secure entrance and exit for safety and unobtrusive security;
- a visitor sleepover facility to enable family contact;
- continuous pathways to help avoid confusion and distress;
- a distinctive high roof to help residents find their way back home.

(Habell, 2010; Northern Housing Consortium, 2010; Stockdale, 2010)

GETTING HOUSING AND THE BUILT ENVIRONMENT ONTO THE WELLBEING AGENDA

The government's recent document, *New Horizons, Confident Communities, Brighter Futures* (HM Government, 2010), provides an evidence base to support the argument for housing as a positive factor in the wellbeing agenda to help inform local plans and commissioning priorities. The document reiterates the fundamental importance of housing for wellbeing and social cohesion.

There is a range of statutory and non-statutory regimes whereby the wellbeing agenda can be enhanced at the local level. For example, the Local Government Act 2000 provides the power for LAs to promote and improve the economic, social and environmental wellbeing of their areas. In addition, the more recent Local Government and Public Involvement Act 2007 required the then PCTs and LAs to produce a Joint Strategic Needs Assessment (JSNA) of the current and future health and wellbeing of their local community, including stakeholders, working with communities themselves and identifying links to other strategies. This process also helps to inform LAA priorities and targets to improve service commissioning, to improve health outcomes and to reduce inequalities (DH, 2007). It is also important that the JSNA aligns closely to the LSP, the Sustainable Community Strategy and other allied interventions.

It is important that all tenures of housing and wellbeing form part of the JSNA, so that appropriate and enhanced services can be commissioned. This helps pool data from different local actors, including housing, social care, health services and others, to provide a more thorough picture of what is currently being delivered and where there may still be gaps in service provision. Many useful examples of how partnership working between housing and care services has been effectively integrated can be found in Davis *et al.* (2009).

To be successful and sustainable, those involved in housing and wellbeing need to help ensure that these areas become a routine part of the resource allocation process. There is a range of ways in which this might be done. To be successful and sustainable in health promotion, JSNA must focus on the socioeconomic determinants of health and this is where housing plays a fundamental role. The links to housing, safety and health are well established and JSNA provide an opportunity for those working in housing to promote housing and wellbeing across tenures, such as in making the case for fuel poverty (affordable warmth) to be included in the private housing sector, which proves particularly hard to reach, or in tackling temporary accommodation, particularly for children.

The organisations that have been most successful in getting housing onto public health and wellbeing agendas within partnerships have been those that have demonstrated a sound local evidence base for their strategies and interventions. The Housing Health and Safety Rating System (HHSRS) has proven particularly useful for this task, and subsequent work such as the introduction of the HHSRS cost calculator has helped housing practitioners to demonstrate the cost-effectiveness of their work in areas such as alleviating fuel poverty and reducing the risk of home accidents for older people, or improving domestic security and therefore the feeling of being safe in one's home, by sometimes relatively inexpensive adaptations that have a positive effect on wellbeing (Davidson *et al.*, 2009).

CONCLUSION

The importance of housing and the built environment to wellbeing cannot be overstated. A person's home, its location and subsequent relationships within the community provide the basis for physical and mental health and wellbeing status. The design of the built environment is fundamental to how people use and enjoy the environment they occupy. Those living in a decent home in a well thought-through local setting with good amenities, facilities and services stand a greater chance of a better quality of life. However, the wellbeing agenda is seriously hampered by the many households living in non-decent and otherwise unsatisfactory housing in deprived local environments, and low levels of social capital and capacity. In addition, the changing needs of our growing elderly population provide emerging challenges for policy makers. As housing and the built environment are so fundamental to both health and quality of life, they must take their places at the top of the wellbeing agenda.

Activity 15.1

1. Identify the ways in which your organisation has actively promoted the role of housing and/or the built environment and wellbeing through established partnerships to meet a specific identified need.

- Who argued the case for housing and/or the built environment and wellbeing;
- through which forum;
- what local and national evidence was used;
- who 'championed' the process and why;
- how successful was the process and how long-lived?

2. How would you define the difference between 'housing and health' and 'wellbeing and housing'? Why might it matter? Give real or hypothetical examples.

Further reading and websites

Commission for Architecture and the Built Environment (CABE) available at **www.designcouncil.org.uk/our-work/cabe/www.cabe.org.uk**

CABE seeks to improve quality of life through design, advising on well-designed buildings, places and spaces. It produces a range of good quality, accessible literature on wellbeing, sustainability, independent living, inclusion, etc., including case studies.

Chartered Institute of Environmental Health available at **www.cieh.org**

The professional award-giving and campaigning body leading on environmental and public health, producing a range of publications and other guidance.

Chartered Institute of Housing available at **www.cih.org**

Supports housing professionals to maximise community wellbeing and produces a range of publications.

Department of Health available at **www.dh.gov.uk/en/index.htm**

Much good-quality, accessible literature on wellbeing, sustainability, independent living, inclusion etc., including case studies.

Department for Communities and Local Government available at **www.communities.gov.uk**

Produces a range of useful publications concerned with local governance, housing, planning, the environment, etc.

Housing Learning and Improvement Network available at **http://www.housinglin.org.uk**

This network is concerned with integration and whole system reform, housing with care, assistive technology and partnership working, and promotes innovative housing, care and support solutions for older and vulnerable people, developing models and best practice.

Chapter 16

Education and Wellbeing

Bill Goddard

Learning outcomes

In this chapter you will learn how to:

- appreciate the range of wellbeing issues that need to be addressed in education;

- discuss what is being done by schools and local authorities to address staff needs, as well as the needs of children and students;

- explain how the school curriculum is being developed in order to embrace wellbeing as a key part of the curriculum.

This chapter focuses on wellbeing and education. It provides an overview and some background to the issues that are addressed in education, particularly in schools, although some consideration is also given to Further and Higher Education. There is a clear indication of the statutory requirements from which the need to focus on wellbeing is based, and within the chapter there are examples of how the issues are addressed by schools and local authorities.

INTRODUCTION

In this chapter, wellbeing will be addressed in relation to schools, children, school staff, parents and governors, as well as Further and Higher Education students and staff. There will be some discussion relating to the meaning and understanding of wellbeing, as well as consideration of the range of influential documents that underpins the idea of wellbeing in education.

In addition to theoretical perceptions of the nature of wellbeing, there will also be real-life examples of how the notion of wellbeing is put into practice. There are a range of interweaving factors that are important aspects of the idea of wellbeing and they encompass government documents, academic research, local authority perspectives, the Office for Standards in Education (OFSTED), and real examples from real institutions.

The chapter will address key drivers in terms of schools, namely the Every Child Matters (ECM) agenda, and Social and Emotional Aspects of Learning (SEAL). These two key developments could be said to be the primary drivers that underpin the development of wellbeing awareness in schools.

WHAT DO WE MEAN BY WELLBEING IN AN EDUCATIONAL CONTEXT?

Section 38(1) of the 2006 Education and Inspections Act defines wellbeing in terms of the matters mentioned in section 10(2) of the Children Act 2004, which are:

- physical and mental health and emotional wellbeing;
- protection from harm and neglect;
- education, training and recreation;
- the contribution made by the pupil to society;
- social and economic wellbeing.

In these terms, wellbeing relates to the five *Every Child Matters* (2005) outcomes that children should be healthy, stay safe, enjoy and achieve, make a positive contribution and enjoy economic wellbeing. These provide the basis for inspections by OFSTED.

However, in 2008 Ereaut and Whiting conducted research for the Department for Children, Schools and Families (DCSF) in which they identified significant ambiguity around the definition, use and function of the word 'wellbeing', not only in government circles but also in the wider world. They assert that the term is a cultural construct that represents a shifting set of meanings, seeming to relate to a collective agreement among groups of people as to what makes a 'good life'. They noted that the term seemed to change meaning over time and that they had identified evidence that showed the use of the term, in 2008 at least, was unstable. The outcome they expressed relating to this was that the Department needed a deliberate strategy to manage its position within the ambiguity and instability (Ereaut and Whiting, 2008). The research report provides a significant linguistic analysis of the origins, use and development of the term 'wellbeing', as well as providing a comprehensive list of online sources that relate to the understanding of the meaning of the word.

Warnick (2009) examined the term wellbeing in relation to its use by Harry Brighouse in his book *On Education*. Warnick's analysis appeared in the journal *Theory and Research in Education* under the title 'Dilemmas of autonomy and happiness'. In this paper he identifies that Brighouse had discussed in his book the place of human flourishing in liberal educational theory and that he had linked this idea to a psychological concept of 'subjective wellbeing'. It is asserted that social scientists gauge this concept through measures of self-reported life satisfaction, depression and anxiety, and positive emotions. It is also clear from this paper that a connection has been made between subjective wellbeing, human flourishing and happiness. As a whole, this paper examines the notion of subjective wellbeing and within its analysis it raises questions about connected ideas of happiness, autonomy, economic participation, truth, critical reflection, the discernment of propaganda and error, and the capacity to arrive at a realistic picture of life. As in the Ereaut and Whiting (2008) research, what becomes clear is that there is no clear definition of the word 'wellbeing' or of its implications in terms of education, and that effectively this is a living construct that is certainly high profile at the present time. As Warnick (2009) notes in relation to those interconnected ideas mentioned above, it is not clear where social science research in this area may lead, but there are areas where further work may throw more light on what wellbeing means and what its implications are for education.

In 2007, White discussed wellbeing and education in terms of issues of culture and authority. As an educational philosopher, his paper follows a similar route to Brighouse. He begins by saying that there is a need to explicate the concept of personal wellbeing and that 'a personally fulfilling life is one largely filled with successful and wholehearted engagement in intrinsically worthwhile activities' (White, 2007, p. 18). He wonders if wellbeing is objectively determinable and if so, how? White (2007) notes that our wellbeing is built around things that we can do and experience, and that this parallels morality in that wellbeing depends on our culture and cultural change. He also relates this approach to the recent work of Howard Gardner on *Multiple Intelligences* (Gardner, 1983) and of Edmund Holmes (Holmes, 1911), who discussed education in terms of self-realisation and as based on six instincts – the communicative, dramatic, artistic, musical, inquisitive and constructive.

Throughout the various accounts discussing the meaning of wellbeing, the idea of happiness recurs, particularly through the work of Richard Layard (Layard, 2005). Generally the idea is treated cautiously by other writers, possibly since it seems difficult to quantify either the nature or experience of happiness. Nevertheless, the idea of happiness recurs and it is easy to see on a simple level how the enjoyment of learning – being happy – can contribute to real learning.

Previously, in 2002, Konu and Rimpelä considered a conceptual model of wellbeing in schools. In their model, wellbeing is connected with teaching and education, and with learning and achievements. Indicators of wellbeing are divided into four categories: school conditions (having), social relationships (loving), means for self-fulfilment (being) and health status. They relate the development of wellbeing to the WHO health-promoting school programme and also the coordinated school health programme in the USA. Their model is based on Allardt's (1976) sociological theory of welfare and assesses wellbeing as an entity in the school setting. As other authors have noted, Allardt indicates that wellbeing is something that is defined historically and is then redefined when living conditions change. It seems to be about the satisfaction of basic needs. Konu and Rimpelä (2002) have used this model to develop their own school wellbeing model, a model that connects teaching, education and learning with wellbeing. In terms of wellbeing, the key characteristics that they believe have to be considered embrace elements of having, loving, being and health. In real terms these can be interpreted so that having relates to school conditions, loving to social relationships, being to the means for self-fulfilment, and health to health status.

SCHOOLS

School governing bodies have been under a duty to promote the wellbeing of children and young people, in terms of the five *Every Child Matters* outcomes, since September 2007.

> Promoting the wellbeing of children and young people is at the heart of the mission of the 21st century school and the wellbeing guidance will capture and support the enthusiasm of Schools to fulfil this role. (DCSF, 2005)

Furthermore it was stated that:

> wellbeing is more than pleasant emotions, it is a positive and

sustainable condition that allows individuals, groups or nations to thrive and flourish ... (DCSF, 2005)

In October 2008 the government made a commitment to making Personal, Social, Health and Economic education (PSHE) a statutory subject within the National Curriculum, making clear its intention to enhance the role of the school in promoting children's wellbeing. In light of this, the National Children's Bureau (NCB) made 'Wellbeing in Schools' a policy priority for the academic year 2008/9. In doing this it campaigned for:

- support for school leaders to implement ECM;
- enabling school governors to promote wellbeing, including young people's development of life skills;
- ensuring effective implementation and delivery of statutory PSHE;
- monitoring wellbeing in schools;
- reforming school inspection and school improvement in line with ECM;
- developing and promoting participative approaches to learning and teaching. (NCB, 2008, p. 1)

It is worth noting that the NCB was already constructing a programme about wellbeing from birth.

As we have seen, the ECM agenda was established by the government in 2004 and essentially required that attention should be given by schools to the following five areas in terms of their pupils:

- be healthy;
- stay safe;
- enjoy and achieve;
- make a positive contribution;
- achieve economic wellbeing.

Statutorily, the Children Act (2004) required that attention be given to physical and mental health and wellbeing, protection from harm and neglect, education, training and recreation, the making of a positive contribution to society, and social and economic wellbeing. Ultimately, of course, the intention behind these developments was the improvement of performance of schools and children. These were supported by a curriculum resource produced by the DCSF in 2005, which was aimed at helping primary schools develop children's social, emotional and behavioural skills. The resource was called *Social and Emotional Aspects of Learning (SEAL): improving behaviour, improving learning*. The advice contained seven themes and was intended to be used by schools that had identified the social and emotional aspects of learning as a key focus. It was developed over two years in over 500 schools who took part in the Primary National Strategy's Behaviour and Attendance pilot. The themes were:

- new beginnings;
- getting on and falling out;
- say no to bullying;
- going for goals;
- good to be me;
- relationships;
- changes.

The audience for this guidance included school governors, head teachers and teaching assistants, as well as teachers and parents, and the aim of the material was to develop underpinning qualities and skills that help to promote positive behaviour and effective learning. Its focus was on five social and emotional aspects of learning: self-awareness, managing feelings, motivation, empathy and social skills. The materials were intended to help children develop skills such as understanding another's point of view, working in a group, sticking at things when they get difficult, resolving conflict and managing worries. They built on work already in place in many schools, done through initiatives such as circle time or buddy schemes, and the PSHE and Citizenship curricula.

The combination of ECM and SEAL raised awareness in schools of the need to address aspects of development that relate to wellbeing. Every school has a stated vision, a mission statement and a range of key policies. The ethos of the school is expressed through these policies. The key policies relate to teaching and learning, discipline and behaviour. However, in addition to the teaching and learning activities of the teachers and the teaching assistants, schools also have to interact with and manage their work with a range of outside agencies that bring key knowledge and skills to the school. These include nurses, dental services, educational psychologists, social services, parent support advisers, and language and learning support services. All of these teams of professionals bring expertise to schools in support of pupil learning.

Gutman and Feinstein (2008) conducted research in 2008 into the pupil and school effects of children's wellbeing in primary school, using data from the Avon Longitudinal Study of Parents and Children (ALSPAC). They note that 'whilst there is evidence that schools are important contexts for children's wellbeing, relatively few UK studies have examined school effects (net of family background and wider social and economic factors) on children's wellbeing'. (Gutman and Feinstein, ibid.). In their executive summary they noted that 'the wellbeing and quality of life of children in the UK today are of increasing concern'. They also noted that a recent UNICEF 'report card' ranked the UK in the bottom third of economically advanced nations for child wellbeing (UNICEF, 2007, cited in Gutman and Feinstein, 2008). Their key findings noted that most children experience positive wellbeing in primary school, with some exceptions, and that children's individual experiences of such things as bullying, victimisation and friendships, and their beliefs about themselves and their environment, are the main factors that affect their wellbeing, rather than school-level factors such as the type of school. Only 3 per cent or less of the variation in pupils' mental health and behaviour are attributed to school factors, and these factors are attributed to school disadvantage and school ethos. There were four other key findings:

1. That schools do make a difference to children's wellbeing but it is the children's individual experiences within schools that are important. Interactions between peers and teachers, within the same or different schools, seem to be more important for children's wellbeing than attending a particular school.
2. Socio-demographic factors, with the exception of gender, seem to have no effect on behaviours, although they do affect achievement.
3. Boys have better mental health than girls, believe in their own abilities and feel that they are in control, but they are more likely to engage in anti-social behaviours.
4. Much of the variation in children's wellbeing remains unexplained and the authors suggest that the unmeasured cumulative experiences of children at home and school are important constituents of their overall wellbeing.

Their conclusions assert that patterns of wellbeing begin early in primary school and generally follow a positive path. For that subset of children who display a negative trajectory of wellbeing, they suggest that early identification and intervention may discourage the continuance of a path that may lead to mental health problems, delinquency or school disengagement.

Within the ECM and SEAL agendas there are specific key foci that enable school staff to deliver the wellbeing curriculum. One of these is resilience. Crow (2008) suggests that this is the ability to develop and thrive in adversity and is central to wellbeing. What this refers to is a process that involves a set of protective systems that can counter the effects of adversity. It refers to good outcomes in spite of serious threats to adaptation or development, and works towards the maximum potential that can be achieved. This includes a range of social and parental factors that enable achievement. The challenge faced by schools is how they can enable children to achieve where they do not have the appropriate supporting mechanisms. There is a range of mechanisms that can be embraced in an effort to build resilience in children, and Hart (2008) lists examples as:

- the use of the Healthy Schools Programme and SEAL;
- the involvement of outside agencies in an advisory and supportive role;
- the provision of opportunities to be involved in extracurricular activities;
- the development and maintenance of a strong school ethos of inclusion, equality and cohesion;
- a positive 'can do' approach to problems, encouraging children to increase control over their lives by learning skills such as negotiation, coping and decision making;
- the use of the mass media and the full potential of new technologies;
- providing opportunities for peer support;
- enabling solution-focused approaches, rather then 'learned helplessness'.

As can be seen from the above list, what goes along with the idea of developing resilience is nurture. This is about building confidence and self-esteem, and it can be seen from the ideas suggested above that these characteristics were once developed in children in the home.

Leading for learning

There are multiple discourses of wellbeing ranging from operationalisation, sustainability and holism to philosophical and medical perspectives, and these relate to the range of initiatives that have taken place in schools in recent years. Leading for learning has been a strong focus that has built on the developments of the National College for Leadership of Schools and Children's Services (NCLSCS) and Crow (2008) elaborated on this in an analysis that highlighted wellbeing in terms of 'Leading for Wellbeing' and 'Wellbeing for Learning'. He noted the importance of leadership governance and school culture on the potential positive impact of wellbeing, as well as the need to build sustainable networks to establish a school's contribution to wellbeing outcomes. Interestingly, Crow identifies what wellbeing indicators could be in terms of quantified outcomes over which schools can have significant influence. These quantified outcomes could be based on the perceptions of pupils and parents, and relate specifically to the ECM outcomes and a school's contribution to them. In terms of data-specific indicators, these could be the identification of attendance rates, absenteeism, involvement in PE and sport, take-up of school lunches, rate of permanent exclusions and, in secondary schools, post-16 progression measures.

Perceptions of parents and children are important and, apart from schools providing a range of extracurricular activities, wellbeing may also be seen to embrace opportunities for pupils to contribute to the local community. Potentially it could help pupils of diverse backgrounds to get on well but, of course, it should help pupils to gain the knowledge and skills they will need for their futures. Curriculum choices at the age of 14 need to be broad enough to offer significant opportunities to all pupils, and schools need to use this opportunity for adequate guidance in linking potential study with future career possibilities.

In more instrumental terms, it may be hoped that a focus on wellbeing may promote healthy eating, exercise and a healthy lifestyle and, for younger children, play. It also ought to foster the discouragement of smoking, excess consumption of alcohol and the use of illegal drugs and other harmful substances, in addition to giving good guidance on relationships and sexual health. Programmes ought to help pupils manage their feelings, be resilient, promote equality and counteract discrimination.

What this all means is that children should feel safe and enjoy school. They should feel that they can make good progress, that they are listened to and that they are able to influence decisions in school. They should know about bullying but also about who to approach if they have concerns about this or any other school matter. The personalisation of education for each pupil is clearly expected to embrace these various actions in fostering individual achievement for every child.

Published work on wellbeing in schools

Wellbeing is certainly a focus in schools nowadays and it is also a themed area for discussion at conferences. Apart from the state-maintained sector embracing work focused on wellbeing, as it is required to do, one of the early manifestations of wellbeing in the curriculum can be seen at Wellington School, an independent school in Berkshire. The school has a Head of Wellbeing, Ian Morris, and in 2009 he published his very useful book, *Teaching Happiness and Wellbeing in Schools.* The book provides teachers with a road map that guides the reader through the issues that need to be addressed in wellbeing. We have mentioned them previously in this chapter, but what is really useful for teachers is the extent of the further reading list, ideas for lesson activities, and advice on creating a wellbeing curriculum in a school.

A further useful text is *Education for Social Justice* (2010) by Chapman and West-Burnham, which has the subtitle 'Achieving Wellbeing for All'. This book discusses excellence and equity in education policy and practice, and looks at the role of relationships at many levels. Although the focus seems different to the Morris book, the chapters address the same kinds of issues identified earlier as being key to wellbeing and any wellbeing provision in schools.

Activity 16.1

Identify the key elements of wellbeing related to the ECM agenda and SEAL.

Staff in schools

Attention to wellbeing does not only focus on children. In today's schools there are large numbers of adult staff who perform a multiplicity of roles, from teaching to being a teaching assistant, a technician, administrative support staff and premises management staff, as well as the leadership and management team. Local authorities have taken action to ensure that the adult staff complement in schools is also considered in terms of wellbeing. For instance, at the Wellbeing Programme launch of Essex County Council in September 2009, it was noted that an average of 15 per cent of all teaching staff absences were due to stress: 16 per cent in primary schools, 14 per cent in secondary schools and 12 per cent in special schools. Additionally, on average 11 per cent of support staff absences were also due to stress: 10 per cent in primary, 12 per cent in secondary schools and 12 per cent in special schools. It was noted that stress was listed in the top three reasons for absence. Local authorities also look at their vacancy and turnover data and can identify trends in particular schools or areas. Further discussion, and a case study, regarding this topic can be found in Chapter 17 (Case study 17.3).

FURTHER AND HIGHER EDUCATION STUDENTS AND STAFF

Wellbeing and further education

With regard to Further Education, Maxwell and Warwick (2007) highlighted some ways in which student mental health is being addressed in colleges of Further Education. They conducted a survey of 150 Further Education colleges and interviewed 18 key informants, as well as focusing on five case study colleges. One of the outcomes of this research activity was the suggestion that 'effective promotion of positive mental health and emotional wellbeing was linked to a holistic, multilayered system of support for students' and that this could include:

- personal tutor systems;
- learning support programmes (learning assistants, extra tuition);
- mentors;
- a counselling service;
- health drop-ins (sexual health clinic with a nurse, drugs support drop-in);
- health awareness events (stop smoking initiatives, anti-bullying campaigns);
- group work (on, for example, anger management, relationship violence);
- information about both college and external sources of support (in college diaries, for instance);
- an active student union (organising social events, outings, representing student views to senior management);
- a range of places to spend free time (quiet spaces, student cafés, student common rooms).

(Maxwell and Warwick, 2007, p.1.)

What can immediately be seen from the list above is the similarity of the issues to those that it is thought important to address in schools, some from the primary phase and some more specifically in the secondary phase.

Wellbeing and Higher Education

Wellbeing has also been addressed in the Higher Education sector in recent years. According to the 'Wellbeing' website, which looks at wellbeing in Higher Education, the majority of stakeholders in Higher Education look on wellbeing in broad terms 'encompassing a variety of areas including physical and mental health, management and leadership development, dignity at work, employee communications, health and safety, and occupational health' (HEFCE, 2010). They are of course concerned with students as well as staff. In research undertaken in 2008, the NEF (Steuer and Marks, 2008) note that there is a recognition of the importance of the economic benefits of Higher Education and a need for a holistic approach to wellbeing. It reports research into positive psychology that has shown the importance of the non-economic factors affecting wellbeing. Steuer and Marks report that:

> the authentic experience of positive emotions (such as enjoyment, enthusiasm and interest) enables people to broaden their thought–action repertoires, by being more flexible, seeking out more opportunities and becoming more creative. In addition to their immediate benefits positive experiences help build enduring physical, intellectual and psychological resources (commonly called the broaden-and-build theory of positive emotions). Researchers have highlighted the importance of building relationships with others, encouraging autonomy and reciprocity, supporting people to demonstrate their competences across different domains of life as well as devising strategies that enable people to longer term goals. (Steuer and Marks, 2008, p. 12)

What we can see from these examples from Higher and Further Education is how wellbeing is being considered in both conceptual and practical terms in each arena. The terms of engagement are not dissimilar and neither are they dissimilar from school agendas. The difference in approach is simply one of phase.

Activity 16.2

Identify from National Framework documents, such as ECM and SEAL, the Wellbeing website and the Maxwell and Warwick paper, the key issues that are being addressed by Further and Higher Education institutions in order to ensure the wellbeing of their students and staff.

CONCLUSION

Schools, colleges and universities have been developing in various ways in recent years and successive government initiatives have been focused on raising achievement among school pupils and adult students. School league tables have brought significant stress to schools, and levels of achievement of vocational students in Further Education colleges and of degree classifications of students in universities have been subject to public scrutiny. The concomitant pressures this has brought on pupils, students and staff, as well as parents, have over time led to a realisation that personal wellbeing is of some significant importance.

The summaries in this chapter of the areas of focus that are deemed important provide an outline of those factors that need to be considered in terms of the wellbeing of all those concerned in all phases of education. This is clearly a starting point. Much work is now being developed in schools, colleges and universities, but at this time it is in its earliest phase of development.

Further reading

Barker, R. (ed) (2009) *Making Sense of Every Child Matters – Multi-Professional Practice Guidance*. London: Policy Press

This book examines the implications of the Every Child Matters agenda for working with children.

Cheminais, R. (2008) *How to Achieve the Every Child Matters Standards: a practical guide*. London: Sage

A very useful book that provides a practical resource to help all those involved in working towards the achievement of ECM standards and in delivering positive outcomes for all pupils.

Cheminais, R. (2009) *Effective Multi-Agency Partnerships: putting Every Child Matters into practice*. London: Sage

This book provides a range of practical activities, realistic advice and useful guidance in relation to multiagency approaches and is an important reference work for everyone involved in implementing the ECM agenda.

Chapter 17

Wellbeing and the Workplace

Kate Beaven-Marks, Anneyce Knight and
Bill Goddard

Learning outcomes

In this chapter you will learn how to:

- understand international issues and applications;

- understand UK government policy relating to occupational
  wellbeing;

- consider applications and effects of wellbeing strategy in the
  workplace.

Wellbeing in the workplace is an extensive topic. For the purposes of
this chapter, government policy relating to occupational wellbeing is
explored and three examples of wellbeing in the workplace in the UK
are discussed in detail: wellbeing in the NHS, wellbeing in Higher
Education and wellbeing within teaching, together with a case study
providing some insight into wellbeing in China.

INTRODUCTION

Wellbeing as a concept has a long history associated with the WHO
definition of health made in 1948. Subsequently, there have been
several prominent international conferences, including the Alma Ata
Primary Care Conference in 1978, Ottawa (1986), Adelaide (1988),
Sundsvall (1991), Jakarta (1997), Mexico (2000) and Bangkok (2005).
Each conference has focused on strengthening health promotion policy,
principles and practice and creating health alliances.

The WHO 'Global Strategy for Health for All by the Year 2000' initiative, launched in 1981 following the Alma Ata conference in the then USSR, was addressed by the Ottawa conference in 1986, and led to the Ottawa Charter for Health Promotion. The Charter promoted the enabling of people to increase control over and improve their health, and saw health promotion as being beyond just the health sector and as also including healthy lifestyles and wellbeing. The Charter considers that the fundamentals for good health are: a sustainable ecosystem and sustainable resources; education; food; income; peace; shelter; and social justice and equity. Furthermore, three strategies were identified for health promotion, those of 'Advocate', 'Mediate' and 'Enable'. These initiatives inform wellbeing policies, strategies and models around the world, including the UK.

Case study 17.1 Wellbeing in China

In China, as the economy develops quickly, personal wellbeing has been given a great deal of attention by the government, society and health institutions. The ways to promote wellbeing are quite diverse and multifaceted, as wellbeing depends not only on factors such as physiology, psychology and outlook on life but also on the interaction of many individual factors as well, such as the social and natural environment (macro-environment) and the workplace environment (micro-environment).

The government mainly takes care of building a good social environment and the natural environment (such as the development of labour policy, health policy, social insurance policy, environmental policy). Social organisations focus on implementing these policies in different ways. For example, public health agencies have set up a good medical network in charge of finding and monitoring workplace environmental hazards. The public health agencies also administer workers' periodic physical check-ups and provide health education to different worker groups within their working environment in order to prevent and control disease such as, for example, HIV and epidemics such as SARS. The environment agency is responsible for monitoring air, water, climate, and even micro-environments such as workshops, in order to improve further the labour environment and wellbeing conditions and reduce occupational risks. Social welfare agencies provide allowances for health and improve medical insurance. News agencies via the media (television, newspapers, radio, etc.) provide a wide range of health education, which includes promoting physical exercise, explaining about traditional medicine and health, psychological interviews, enhancing the family network and working relationships, treatment and legal counselling. The private sector has begun to intervene in health programmes such as health promotion, physical exercise and psychological counselling. The citizens themselves have started to learn self-care methods for physical and mental health, to learn how to face and deal with social relations at home and in the workplace, and how to access the facilities when suffering from mental and physical problems. But are these enough? To improve human wellbeing, a lot of things need to be discussed and a variety of methods explored in a society that is developing all the time.

With thanks to Dr Jane Liu, Director Medical Care and Health Education Centre, United International College (Beijing Normal University, Hong Kong Baptist University), Zhuhai, China

In the UK, the 2005 strategy from the Department of Health (DH), Department for Work and Pensions (DWP) and the Health and Safety Executive (HSE), entitled *Health, Work and Wellbeing: caring for our future*, is a strategy for the health and wellbeing of working-age people. It was published at a time when it could be considered that the focus was on ill health. The aims of the strategy focused on:

1. helping people manage minor health problems at work;
2. helping people return to health following an absence from work because of illness;
3. helping people avoid work-related ill-health problems.

(DH *et al.*, 2005)

The report indicated that there would be 'leading by example', with the NHS, government and local authorities becoming exemplars of healthy workplaces.

Working for a Healthier Tomorrow

In March 2008 the focus moved more clearly to health and wellbeing. Dame Carol Black's review on the health of Britain's working-age population, *Working for a Healthier Tomorrow* (Black, 2008), looked at the human, social and economic costs of impaired health and wellbeing, specifically in relation to working life in Britain. Her review aimed to consider barriers to good health and interventions to promote good health, and that included services and changes in attitudes, behaviours and practices, as well as looking at expanding the role for occupational health to provide a broad collaborative and multidisciplinary service.

Research specifically commissioned for the review found 'considerable evidence' of the economic benefits of health and wellbeing programmes (Black, 2008, p. 10). Waddell and Burton (2006) are cited in Black (2008, p. 124) as having concluded that work was generally good for both physical and mental health and wellbeing (Black, 2008, p. 21). The vision outlined in Black's review focused on three primary objectives:

* prevention of illness and promotion of health and wellbeing;
* early intervention;
* an improvement in the health of those out of work.

At the time of the review there was a working-age population of 36.6 million people, with a further million people working beyond the state pension age and almost 75 per cent of working-age people in employment (Black, 2008, p. 29). South Ribble Borough Council are quoted in the review as saying, 'most people in employment spend 60 per cent of their waking hours in work ... the workplace is a great place to promote the benefits of enjoying a healthy, active lifestyle' (Black, 2008, p. 51). It is clear that the workplace is an ideal environment in which to influence the workforce with health and wellbeing information, education and support.

Activity 17.1

Consider an organisation that you have worked for or currently work for. How does it promote your wellbeing? What is the impact of this promotion on you?

Perhaps also of interest is the definition of wellbeing given in the review, referencing Waddell and Burton's (2006) description: 'wellbeing is the subjective state of being healthy, happy, contented, comfortable and satisfied with one's quality of life. It includes physical, material, social, emotional ("happiness"), and development and activity dimensions' (Black, 2008, p. 124).

In response to the Black review, the government's *Improving Health and Work: Changing Lives*, presented by the DWP and the DH, was published on 25 November 2008 and indicated aspirations for:
* creating new perspectives on health and work;

- improving work and workplaces;
- supporting people to work.

(DWP and DH, 2008)

Key initiatives were identified including the establishment of a Health, Work and Wellbeing Challenge Fund, the appointment of Health, Work and Wellbeing Coordinators from the summer of 2009, and a National Centre for Working-Age Health and Wellbeing (to be established in late 2009). In the appendices of the review, each of Black's recommendations are listed, together with the government action taken, or proposed, for each of the 31 actions identified (DWP and DH, 2008).

The Health, Work and Wellbeing Coordinators have now been appointed and the National Centre for Working Age Health and Wellbeing is currently open for tender and will produce evidence on the impact of occupational health interventions. The Health Work and Wellbeing Challenge Fund is described on the **www.workingforhealth.gov.uk** site as a grant scheme of £4 million over two years from the DWP and it will fund innovative projects for improvements to employee health and welfare.

The Health, Work and Wellbeing Strategy Unit was formed in 2005 and is sponsored by five different government partners: the DWP, DH, HSE, Scottish government and the Welsh assembly. The aim of the unit is to enhance and protect the health and wellbeing of people of working age. The emphasis is on encouraging constructive links between health and work, and the unit seeks to assist more people with health conditions to gain and maintain employment. As part of its cross-organisational nature it draws together a range of partners including employers, trade unions and health care professionals. It also undertakes research on developing the notion that work makes people healthier, especially those who have a health condition and those returning to work following a period of unemployment. The Unit's website **www.dwp.gov.uk/health-work-and-well-being/about-us** offers a range of tools, guidance and practical advice.

WELLBEING IN THE NHS

As Europe's largest employer and one of the world's largest employers, the NHS could be seen to be leading by example on health and wellbeing. In response to Dame Carol Black's review (Black, 2008) on the health of the UK's working-age population, Dr Steve Boorman, an expert in occupational health, was appointed to lead the independent NHS Health and Wellbeing Review, which had been announced by Secretary of State

Alan Johnson MP on 25 November 2008. The review would consider existing evidence and good practice for working-age people in general and for the NHS workforce specifically. It is also interesting to note that *The NHS Constitution* of March 2010 (NHS, 2010) demonstrates commitments to the health and wellbeing of all NHS staff, pledging support and opportunities for staff on wellbeing, health and safety.

An interim report was first produced (NHS, 2009a), which identified a range of actions and considered that the overarching point is that wellbeing needs to be recognised as a 'crucial issue' at board level as much as at ward level (NHS, 2009b, p. 5). Responsibility is considered to belong to every single member of staff. However, it identified that 'making this happen requires nothing less than a sea change in the way in which staff health and wellbeing is perceived' (NHS, 2009a, p. 5). The report goes on to discuss the strong business case for investing in health and wellbeing. Using the NHS as an example, with the potential for reducing sickness absence rates by one-third, 33.4 million additional work days would be saved, an estimated annual direct cost saving of £555 million (NHS, 2009a, p. 6).

The NHS is to be applauded for its openness with regard to supporting materials for the interim report. It is possible to download the call for evidence, staff perception surveys and equality impact assessment on **www.nhshealthandwellbeing.org/InterimReport.html** It is also possible to download the detailed literature review (Hassan *et al.*, 2009). The literature review's aims were to:

1. examine the extent of poor health and wellbeing in British workplaces and the NHS;
2. review the scholarly literature on the effectiveness of health workplace interventions;
3. identify lessons from good practice comparators.

The literature review highlights the lack of consensus among academics regarding the definition of wellbeing and referred to both Danna and Griffin (1999) (cited in Hassan *et al.*, 2009) and Warr (1999) (cited in Hassan *et al.*, 2009). Danna and Griffin (1999) consider wellbeing to be broader than health, and Warr (1999) offered a distinction between workplace wellbeing and personal, or 'context free', wellbeing.

The literature review findings indicated that poor health and wellbeing at work was having significant societal, economic, organisational and personal consequences and that health and wellbeing in the workplace are particular challenges for the NHS. Therefore, three approaches, physical, psychological and societal consequences, were explored by the literature review, which considered health, wellbeing and work; effectiveness of workplace interventions; and identifications of good practice.

Prior to publication of the final report, a period of consultation with stakeholders took place. At these events, held across the country, opinions were sought and many of the recommendations were included in the final report. The final report (NHS, 2009b) emphasised that wellbeing is more than just the absence of disease, but is also concerned with achieving mental, physical and social contentment. It can be noted that this complements the WHO's Constitution referred to at the beginning of this chapter. Recommendations of the final report include improving organisational behaviours and performance, providing the necessary services, and embedding health and wellbeing in systems and infrastructures. Separate to the final report, the staff health and wellbeing case studies (NHS, 2009c) were also published, giving good practice examples of 50 NHS organisations and nine non-NHS organisations from the government, private sector and academia.

Case study 17.2

Example one: The Airedale NHS Trust (stepped care)

At the Airedale NHS Trust the adoption of a three-pronged approach to mental health in the workplace, with prevention, retention and rehabilitation, and with early CBT (Cognitive Behaviour Therapy), brief, highly structured counselling and complementary therapy services, had a proactive as well as a reactive approach unlike their previously reactive service. There was a significant reduction in sickness absence rates to little over 5 per cent, increased employee morale and reduced staff turnover (NHS, 2009c, pp. 2–4).

Example two: NHS Knowsley – Knowsley Health and Wellbeing

A partnership between NHS Knowsley and the Knowsley Metropolitan Borough Council set up a workforce health programme. A key element of the programme was the 'Fitbug', which is a pedometer. Significantly, 67 per cent of all participants considered using Fitbug helped change their lifestyle: 71 per cent of all participants were now walking more to work and 76 per cent of all participants were walking more outside work. Furthermore, they reported that one of their most successful outcomes for 2007/8 was the uptake of complementary therapies, with evidence of an improvement in staff morale. Overall sickness rates fell to under 5 per cent in March 2008 (NHS, 2009c, pp. 26–7).

Overall, the case histories reflected a range of provisions, from healthy eating to fitness programmes, counselling, CBT and complementary therapies, together with a range of early intervention strategies.

WELLBEING IN HIGHER EDUCATION

The Royal College of Psychiatrists (RCP) considers in its report on *The Mental Health of Students in Higher Education* (RCP, 2003) that Higher Education makes significant provisions for the wellbeing of students. From a student services perspective, the student services organisation, the Association of Managers of Student Services in Higher Education (AMOSSHE), informs and supports leaders of student services. It represents and promotes the student experience and the promotion and the development and sharing of good practice in student services. Its financial report of February 2009 (AMOSSHE, 2009) indicates the importance of services to underpin learning, development and wellbeing, and these are reported to be of increasing importance to both the quality of the student experience and to the 'distinctiveness in graduate outcomes' (point 2.2.1), with wellbeing learning opportunities available more diversely than simply in the classroom (point 3.5), such as, for example, in the residence halls and student union bars.

The main report of the Higher Education Funding Council for England (HEFCE) 2010 considers that employee wellbeing programmes in Higher Education Institutions (HEI) offer support to help maintain commitment and motivation and, to quote from Dame Carol Black's *Working for a Healthier Tomorrow* (Black, 2008), that while many employers are uncertain of the business case for wellbeing investment, the 2008 review indicated that 'good health is good business' (HEFCE, 2010, p. 109). The report goes on to refer to a case study of employee wellbeing at the University of Brighton (HEFCE, 2010, p. 109), which indicated that following interventions including CBT, counselling and welfare advice, sickness absence levels for staff have fallen each year over the past three years.

The 2007/8 HEFCE project Creating Success through Wellbeing in Higher Education aimed to share best practice, facilitate networking and support staff wellbeing in the HE sector, and it has been followed by a two-year HEFCE-funded project called Improving Employee Performance through Wellbeing and Engagement. The project has major stakeholders from the health and safety and occupational health fields, including the chair of the University Safety and Health Association (USHA). Key actions include wellbeing surveys, workplace interventions and sharing of information. The project website, **www.wellbeing.ac.uk**, offers advice, guidance, information and resources to support the aim of the project, which is to take HEIs to the next level in their understanding and practice relating to employee engagement and wellbeing.

When considering wellbeing in the HE sector, the *Times Higher Education*, in an article on 21 January 2010 'Get happy, get on with it' (*Times Higher Education*, 2010), refers to the PriceWaterhouseCooper 2008 report *Building the Case for Wellness*, which calculates a return of £4.17 for every £1 spent on staff wellbeing (PriceWaterhouseCooper, 2008, p. 6). This report, commissioned as part of Dame Carol Black's review to investigate the wider business case for workplace wellbeing, reported that workplace wellness makes commercial sense, with wellness programmes having positive impacts on intermediate (non-financial) and bottom-line (financial) benefits such as reduced sickness absence, leading to reduced overtime payments and less temporary recruitment.

The *Times Higher Education* (2010) article also comments on the efforts of some universities, including Leeds and Bristol. Leeds and Bristol universities are now to work in partnership and consider various aspects of wellbeing in the workplace, such as how to engage and support their staff to perform better during challenging times. On its website, Leeds University has also recently announced a £350 000 HEFCE award to continue to build the evidence for relationships between wellbeing and staff engagement (Leeds University, 2010a). Leeds University has a wellbeing strategy for stakeholders including staff, students and other university members. Its wellbeing strategy's direction (Leeds University, 2010b) is formed by the Ottawa Charter and the DWP's Health, Work and Wellbeing Strategy (Dame Carol Black's review of the working-age population and workplace health and wellbeing frameworks). Gary Tideswell, Director of Wellbeing, Safety and Health at Leeds University, and Kim Shutler presented a paper, 'Leading Transformational Change' (Tideswell and Shutler, 2009), at the HEFCE and the Leadership Foundation Conference 'Leadership Governance and Management Projects' in 2009, presenting a case study on their wellbeing work at the University of Leeds and examples from other universities. Tideswell emphasised there is a clear business benefit to the work they do, citing a wellness management pilot for staff which resulted, for one of the three test groups, in a decrease of absence levels of 1.6 days per person per year.

WELLBEING IN EDUCATION

Contractually, and arising from the National Workload Agreement, the Teachers' Pay and Conditions document includes a requirement that all teachers should enjoy a reasonable life/work balance. This puts specific responsibilities on head teachers in respect of their staff, and a similar duty is placed on governing bodies in respect of head teachers. In addition to this, the *Green Book* (conditions of service for local government staff) also requires a commitment to maintaining a reasonable life/work balance. There is also a common law and legal duty regarding the health and welfare of employees under health and safety legislation and working time regulations. Achieving life/work balance may embrace a consideration of such matters as flexible working, flexible absence, an acceptable working culture, appropriate provision of facilities and benefits, and also recognition of the need to pursue personal interests outside working time. When such considerations are taken account of in a proactive and positive manner, there are significant benefits to be gained, such as the provision of a motivated and committed workforce, improved recruitment and retention, reduced absenteeism, a more productive and focused workforce, and a greater flexibility in order to meet demands.

Medway Council includes a page on its council website that addresses staff wellbeing in schools. It is interesting that its first comments relate to the comments above, in that it says 'as many schools have faced problems in recruiting and retaining staff, the need for a proactive approach to staff wellbeing has become apparent. Investing in staff health and wellbeing will contribute directly to more efficient organisational performance, improved staff morale and motivation, all of which help drive school improvement' (Medway Council, 2010). The page goes on to say that:

the aims of Medway Council's wellbeing programme are to:

- promote supportive and well-informed managerial practice, which actively develops healthy workplaces, focusing on organisational progress;
- enable staff, as individuals and in groups, to manage the pressures they face successfully;
- use a range of evaluation methods to identify strengths and weaknesses;

- measure progress systematically to inform future action;
- provide a means of sharing information and research about best practice.

The wellbeing programme underpins the Workforce Reform agenda, performance management and professional development opportunities for all staff working in schools that buy this service. (Medway Council, 2010)

The council identifies potential hazards in terms of culture, demands, control, role, change, relationships and support, and also identifies a range of both individual and organisational symptoms of stress, with their potential negative outcomes. As we can see from the web pages, this is an outline of a wellbeing service approach that Medway Council hopes schools will buy into.

Teacher wellbeing

Briner and Dewberry conducted a research study in 2007 into the links between staff wellbeing and school performance, and concluded that, if the improvement of school performance is a key aim, there is a need to pay attention to teacher wellbeing. They note that 'happier, motivated teachers may make pupils feel happier, motivated and more confident. Happier teachers may also be able to concentrate better on the job of teaching, and experience more motivation to help pupils in need of special attention' (Briner and Dewberry, 2007, p. 4). They also concluded that it was most likely that there was a two-way relationship between teachers and pupils in terms of wellbeing and performance, and that this can lead either to a virtuous circle or a downward spiral, both dependent on teacher wellbeing and potentially concomitant responses in pupil performance.

Case study 17.3 Wellbeing project in East Sussex

Over a period of time, one school in East Sussex has put in place initiatives to address some aspects of staff wellbeing:

- quickly attending to problems like photocopiers not working;
- updating all staff toilets;
- increasing car park spaces;
- installing machines dispensing free tea and coffee in the staff room;
- an extra dishwasher;
- one member of staff is paid for 15 minutes, three times a day, to ensure that clean cups are available at the start of every break and lunch time;
- a free fleece with school logo for each member of staff (beneficial for playground duty on chilly days);
- free tee shirts, overalls, etc. provided to the caretaker;
- proper attention is always paid to staff farewells, the head teacher always attends and all staff members who are leaving are properly thanked and their achievements and contribution to the school acknowledged through, for example, whole-school end-of-term assemblies;
- a summer barbecue for all staff, paid for from school fund;
- the establishment of a staff welfare fund to pay for flowers and cards in cases of sickness and other absences;
- when staff are absent because of long-term illness, there is an expectation that colleagues will visit;
- there is some limited flexibility about time off during term time, in case of exceptional circumstances;
- staff in job-share posts have a degree of freedom to negotiate their working arrangements between them, allowing for greater flexibility;
- a staff Christmas lunch every year, in school, paid for by school;
- a staff Christmas evening out, subsidised by school;
- on inset days, part-time and job-share staff are paid to attend if the inset does not fall on their usual working day;
- resources have been put in to ensure that the staff room is a comfortable, relaxing place for all members of the team.

With thanks to Corinne McGregor, Deputy Head Teacher, All Saints Church of England Primary School, Bexhill-on-Sea.

CONCLUSION

The government is responding to increasing awareness of wellbeing in the workplace by conducting reviews and responding with initiatives and objectives. Evidence from a range of sources, including the Black Review, the NHS, the PriceWaterhouseCooper review and HEFCE, clearly indicate that in some areas the support for wellbeing interventions is clear. It would also seem that the economic business case is being clearly made that health and wellbeing interventions can pay off. Furthermore, a simple internet search on wellbeing will locate information, services, resources and signposts to more. However, it is not yet clear whether there is sufficient evidence of positive perceptions of wellbeing's importance. Benefits of and accessibility to wellbeing provision in all workplaces, particularly smaller and medium-sized organisations, are required and may benefit from further investigation to create strategies and to offer a more targeted approach. This suggests that perhaps more could be made of the 'Working for Health' website at the ground level and that health and social care students and professionals should explore wellbeing in the workplace in more detail.

Further reading

Rath, T. and Harter, J. (2010) *Wellbeing: the five essential elements*. New York: Gallup Press

This book discusses five essential elements (career, social, financial, physical and community) of wellbeing, with career wellbeing identified as the most essential.

Kinder, A., Hughes, R. and Cooper, C.L. (2008) *Employee Wellbeing Support: a workplace resource*. West Sussex: Wiley and Sons

An edited compilation of expert contributions that explores the key issues regarding workplace wellbeing.

Chapter 18

Information for Wellbeing

Anne Gill

Learning outcomes

In this chapter you will learn how to:

- understand the role of the media in shaping the public's and health and social care workers' perceptions of health and wellbeing;

- find sources of information on health and wellbeing in the mass media;

- analyse and understand sources of information in the mass media;

- influence the media agenda.

This chapter will examine mass media sources of information on health and wellbeing available to clients and health and social care workers (newspapers, TV, radio and the internet). The chapter will also examine how the perceptions of both public and health care workers, with regard to health and wellbeing, are influenced by the agenda of the media. There will be information on how to analyse and understand information sources and how to influence the media agenda.

INTRODUCTION

A focus on health and wellbeing is an attempt to broaden the definition of care from illness to include quality of life and client empowerment. Changing the definition is only feasible if clients and health and social care workers are able to access and use the best quality health and wellness information.

Health and illness are favourite media themes; they appear in countless news items, documentaries, soap operas and dramas. Images of hospitals, doctors, midwives, other health professionals and patients are constantly flickering on television screens. Tales of wonder drugs and instant cures abound, and can cause disappointment and anger when the reality does not match up or the treatment is not funded.

The concept of wellbeing is not covered by the media in the same way. An internet search using Google News reveals an interesting pattern – news sources are local rather than national newspapers and websites. Reports relate to policies and initiatives rather than cures and scandals and, interestingly, this is the way health professionals would prefer the media to report health care issues in general. However, this approach does have problems in that it is context-dependent and tends to relate to specific conditions like, for example, diabetes and wellbeing, wellbeing for the elderly, etc. Such a focus on specific conditions is helpful for health and social care professionals and sufferers from those conditions, but does not help members of the general public who would like an overall view of the meaning of wellbeing and its application to their lives. The media focus tends to be on events related to health care rather than everyday issues that have an impact on health and wellbeing, and this is clearly demonstrated in an important report from The King's Fund, *Health in the News*, which will be described in detail in the next section.

THE IMPACT OF THE MEDIA ON HEALTH AND SOCIAL CARE ISSUES

Health and social care professionals need to understand how the reporting of health and social issues impacts on the public and influences practice. The following quote from a public health professional in the introduction to The King's Fund report sums up the problem for health- and wellbeing-related issues very well.

> For many of us in public health it often seems that the media focus on health services – particularly their failings – drowns out all comment on health and the daily challenges we face when addressing the health needs of the population. Our experience tells us that what we have to say does not grab the headlines – despite its potential importance in improving health, preventing disease or reducing inequalities. Patterns of media reporting can influence public attitudes and behaviour as well as the priorities of policy makers. If the biggest risks to public health are scarcely

mentioned in the news while stories about NHS waiting times or health scares such as the SARS virus – where health risks to UK health are minimal – regularly make the headlines, it is fair to ask whether the public interest is well served by the media. (King's Fund, 2003, p. 1)

The King's Fund report *Health in the News* is worth quoting in detail, as it sums up the problems for health and social care professionals in promoting wellbeing. Essentially successful attempts are not newsworthy and clients are unlikely to encounter regular stories in the popular press and on television.

Health in the News

The background to the report is that experts in The King's Fund noticed that the media often came to them for information about health services but rarely to seek out information about public health. The questions asked by the report included: 'To what extent did news coverage of health-related issues reflect mortality risks shown in health data? Could and should anything be done about it?' (King's Fund, 2003, p. 2). The report found a general level of dissatisfaction among health professionals regarding the news media, and universal frustration that the power of the media to disseminate information about health issues was being misused.

Media analysis

News programmes on television and radio were examined over a year, and newspapers, both broadsheets and tabloids, were examined for three months. Health issue stories were catalogued and the volume of reporting on risks was compared with the number of deaths attributed to those risks (King's Fund, 2003). Stories fell into two categories: firstly, the NHS – mostly stories about crises such as waiting times or negligence; secondly, health 'scares' – that is, risks to public health that involved little impact on rates of illness and premature deaths. Themes with little coverage included major health risks such as smoking and alcohol, which cause significant amounts of illness and death and impact significantly on wellbeing.

Some news outlets appeared to have particular interests. For example, the BBC's *Ten O'Clock News* carried large numbers of stories about ethical issues in health care, such as the right to die. All the media outlets covered public health issues in features and these often did address issues such as obesity and alcohol, but their good effect is often cancelled out by news headlines that exert a stronger influence on the public (King's Fund, 2003, p. 3).

Does it matter?

It probably does, but public interpretations of what they read or see in the media are so individual that getting evidence for straightforward cause-and-effect relationships is very difficult. The King's Fund report identifies three reasons why it may matter.

First there is evidence that some kinds of media coverage of health issues make an impact on public behaviour; an example of this is the MMR vaccine (the measles, mumps and rubella combined vaccine). The UK is the only country where rates of take-up have dropped. This happened after coverage of one scientific paper linking the MMR jab with autism, so the rate of take-up does appear to be related to media coverage (King's Fund, 2003, p. 4).

Second, the media may be influencing the policy makers. Politicians often assume, not always correctly, that the media is a true reflection of public opinion. They may therefore change current priorities and spending commitments inappropriately when related to the actual health risk (King's Fund, 2003, p. 4).

Third, government priorities influence media agendas in ways that are mutually reinforcing. A good example of this is waiting times. News stories highlight waiting times and the government responds by prioritising waiting times, which therefore encourages the media to find yet more stories. This can spiral out of control, leading the government to invest resources at the expense of other health-related initiatives that bring greater benefits at less cost (King's Fund, 2003, p. 4).

The journalists

When journalists and editors were interviewed some expressed surprise at the patterns of media coverage demonstrated by the content analysis. Most of the reporters and editors rejected the idea of 'proportionality', which implies a close match between the scale of the risk and the weight of reporting, but some were amenable to the idea that news coverage might be more proportionate. The principle behind their refusal of proportionality was that news values are paramount, although they admitted that these are shaped by commercial issues, the priorities of news organisations or, in the case of newspapers, the proprietor. These issues will be addressed later in the chapter.

Activity 18.1

What can we do about public misconceptions of health risks, either as health and social care professionals or wellbeing promoters? The following King's Fund report recommendations make suggestions for what all people involved in health and social care can do to influence the press to report on health and wellbeing issues more responsibly. How would you apply these recommendations to your practice, either via your organisation/workplace or as an individual wellbeing promoter in the community?

The King's Fund recommendations

- A better understanding among public health protagonists about how news is constructed, and the imperatives and constraints under which different news outlets operate.
- Facilitate a better understanding by experts, policy makers and the media of how the public perceive and interpret health risks.
- Stronger advocacy for public health issues at national, regional and local level.
- More skilful presentation of health issues by experts and policy makers for news and features outlets, with attention to the need for accessible language and for sound and pictures for radio and television. (King's Fund, 2003, p. 5).

GETTING THE MESSAGE ACROSS

There are some interesting indications that wellbeing is not following these patterns. In the Google News search mentioned above, topics related to health and wellbeing included teen pregnancies, mental health and a significant proportion of articles about wellbeing and the elderly (Search terms 'health and wellbeing', 25 August 2010). If this focus on real health-related issues is maintained it will have positive implications for the confidence of health and social care professionals in directing clients to media sources, but it also means that much work will be needed to persuade the mass media to focus on issues related to quality of life and promoting health and wellbeing. This next section proposes some strategies that health and social care professionals, and all concerned with health and wellbeing in the community, could use.

Case study 18.1 MMR

One explanation of the MMR 'controversy', which is not really a controversy at all, is the phenomenon of 'false balance'. Balance is an important concept in media coverage of all issues – for example, a balanced approach to reporting is part of the BBC (British Broadcasting Corporation) charter. The convention is that if you present a particular viewpoint you must bring in someone of equal status to oppose that viewpoint. This is ethical journalism with regard to politics and current affairs but it can present problems with science, where the effectiveness and safety of, for example, vaccines and medicines are issues of fact and not opinion, as long as they are supported by the weight of good-quality evidence.

In the MMR 'controversy' there is one paper indicating, not proving, a link between MMR and autism and, on the other side, are the large-scale studies all over the world that have not found a link. No other scientifically verified papers (that is papers that have been published in a reputable journal and been peer reviewed) have found a link between MMR and autism. However, because of the concept of balance and a real desire to act ethically, the media presented the issue as one with an equal weight of opinion on both sides of the argument. Recently, responsible broadcasters and newspapers have attempted to point out that the weight of expert opinion is very much against the existence of a link between MMR and autism but, judging by the continuing reduction in the uptake of MMR vaccine, the public still appears to think that this is a genuine controversy with an equal weight of scientific opinion on both sides of the issue (Department of Health, 2010).

Health and social care issues are sometimes affected by the phenomenon of false balance and it is therefore important for wellbeing promoters to be aware of the importance of an evidence-based approach to the subject and, crucially, to be aware of the difference between evidence and opinion.

Given that the mass media are unlikely to cover wellbeing issues with the same enthusiasm as scandals and crises, it is important that wellbeing promoters are aware of existing mechanisms for promoting their message to the media.

Public relations

Health and social care professionals tend to feel rather helpless when faced with negative images of their specialities and clients in the media. We do not feel we have the skills to influence the media in a positive way, but there are ways to do this by using the principles of public relations. For example, when public relations professionals wish the media to be aware of something they send a press release; they don't wait for reporters to turn up on their doorsteps asking questions. Press releases are an attempt to control the agenda and to persuade the media to print what you wish them to. Of course, this strategy does not always work. If the subject is not on the newspapers' or television's news agenda, even a very well-written press release will not be published, which, for the reasons discussed above, can be a difficulty for health and wellbeing promoters.

It is important to target your press release at the right media outlet. If you work with a small community-based organisation it would not normally be sensible to send press releases to the national media, but news-hungry local papers and free sheets might be very pleased to get a snappy press release regarding a good local initiative. If you work in a Hospital Trust or large health or social care organisation, it will almost certainly have a press office that should be consulted before contacting the media.

Writing a press release

The following points are based on advice from the BBC on writing press releases. General principles for all press releases include:

- Put the key facts first – if they are half way down the page most editors will not even read that far.
- One sheet of A4 – no one reads the second page of a press release.
- Your press release will not be published the next day, so send it well in advance of when you want it to appear – at least two weeks. Press releases are not 'breaking news' regarding startling events. Yours could relate to the launch of a new local strategy to encourage exercise for the elderly, and you will know when it starts. If you have something urgent or startling to relate, use the phone, email or fax.

Essential Information to include on your press release:

- The name of your organisation and contact numbers.
- The date, time, venue and purpose of the event, if appropriate.
- The name and contact number of a person available for interview

(this may be a scary thought but at some point you will need to talk to the press if you want to influence the media agenda).
- Any relevant supplementary information like, for example, the people involved, their qualifications, why the event or initiative is important (supplementary information should be attached to the single-page press release – if the media outlet is going to publish they will read it, if not they won't, but they won't publish without some indication that this is a legitimate venture, and that the people involved have qualifications that match the activity). Don't be influenced by the common view that the media don't check their facts as, in relation to this type of story, they do.

Successful press releases are:

- typed;
- well displayed with key information highlighted, relevant bullet points and spaced paragraphs;
- proof-read – a badly spelt press release will be instantly discarded.

Check you have included everything using the five Ws: Who? What? Where? When? Why?

(Adapted from BBC Radio Nottingham, 2001)

Activity 18.2

We often feel powerless when faced with misrepresentation by the media, but health and social care professionals and related workers are generally well regarded by the public and do have a voice.

1. Choose a current health-related issue that interests you and write a press release, following the above rules.
2. Investigate local newspapers and decide which one it would be best to send it to.
3. Check with the relevant person and send your press release to the chosen newspaper (you never know – it could result in a published story).

Writing and reading news stories, promotional materials and leaflets

You may be involved in both reading and writing for various publications in relation to stories about your specialism, health promotion initiatives, medicines and the various materials promoting health and social care environments.

Writing news stories, promotions and leaflets

When writing news stories, promotions and leaflets, the rules are very similar to those for writing press releases. A good headline is crucial and the main issues and facts should be in the first paragraph. If there is a lot of information to convey, your story may be longer than the one-page press release, but always remember that 'less is more'. Short paragraphs are best and never use a long word when a short one will convey the same meaning. This is not 'talking down' to readers, it is communicating with clarity to a non-specialist audience, but don't go too far in the other direction and use inappropriate street terms or slang. Also ensure your story or promotion has structure – that is, a clearly marked beginning, middle and end.

Most importantly, check the accuracy of your facts. Something as simple as a mistake in an address or phone number will mean that your communication is worthless as you cannot be contacted for advice or comment. Misspellings and grammatical errors will lead to your information being discounted, however important it is. Also, if you are recommending a treatment, diet or exercise regime, you can be held accountable if someone suffers harm and can prove that it relates to the information you have given. If you work in a large organisation there will be procedures to go through before you publish something with the organisation's name on it. Do not use shortcuts and bypass these procedures as they are for your protection as well as for the protection of the organisation. If you are an independent practitioner or voluntary worker, find someone with expertise in the subject to act as a critical friend.

Reading news stories, promotions and leaflets

When you are reading a news story, promotion or leaflet, or watching and listening to television, radio or tracking a story on the web, here are some questions to ask yourself.

What is influencing the messages you are receiving?

In order to answer the above you need to ask some supplementary questions.

- **Which media?** Alan Ginsberg once said 'the medium is the message'. There is some truth in this. For example, television presents news stories in a quite different way to the radio. The language used is different and the use of images predominates on television, whereas radio presenters have to paint verbal pictures. The printed media is different again, with the broadsheets tending towards longer, more thoughtful pieces and the tabloids favouring vivid images with short and easily understood messages. You can apply this to promoting wellbeing, suiting the style to the message. Think about the style you would use if you were writing an advertisement or health promotion leaflet encouraging people to follow particular dietary advice like, for example, 'five vegetable portions a day'. People tend to read these messages in passing, so they remember them if they are short, vivid and easy to understand. It is advisable to use a quite different style for an article for a professional journal on diet and nutrition or for a chapter for a book on wellbeing. Being interviewed on radio or television requires different skills. Presentation styles for these outlets are similar to that for a press release: make sure the main message is conveyed immediately and keep the five Ws – Who? What? Where? When? Why? – firmly in mind.

- **Who owns it?** Regarding the mass media particularly, ownership is probably more important than authorship. The BBC has an enormous range of outlets and is essentially 'owned' and paid for by the nation via the licence fee. It has a commitment to impartiality that is embedded in its charter and is policed by a board of governors. Despite this, the BBC is still accused of bias but it does have to answer these accusations and there are procedures to penalise the organisation if it is found to have broken the rules. Some newspapers are owned by individuals like, for example, Rupert Murdoch. His company owns *The Times* and the *Sun*, as well as Sky television and many other media outlets throughout the world. The Barclay Brothers own the *Telegraph*, Richard Desmond owns the *Express*. Editors of these newspapers insist that they do not allow the owners' views to influence what goes in the paper, but the proprietors choose the editors and tend to choose people who reflect their views. This is important and is influenced by politics and commercial pressures. See the sections below on 'Are commercial pressures influencing the story?' and 'Who is the audience?'

What is the quality of the evidence?

The media are not expected to apply scientific rules of evidence to every story, but there are some basic rules of evidence that they should follow. When presenting a factual report they rely on sources and the rules of evidence mean that the source should ideally be a witness to the event, not relying on hearsay. The role of the expert witness is more complicated. Health and social care professionals and health and wellbeing promoters may be regarded as expert witnesses in their specialisms. The media will generally check that the expert is qualified so that, for example, if an expert is titled as doctor, nurse or therapist, they will check that the qualification is genuine and that the individual can legitimately discuss, for example, diet or exercise. However, they would not feel it was necessary to follow the rules of the scientific community and wait for independent validation, which is why dubious health-related stories often appear in the media.

Are commercial pressures influencing the story?

Apart from the BBC, all newspapers, radio and television stations exist to make money. Even the BBC has to justify its licence fee by producing good audience figures for its programmes. Commercial pressures affect the interpretation of the news and stories have to sell newspapers. The perception is that human interest stories sell best. Rather than a dry statistics-based article about accident and emergency waiting times, the media much prefer a story based on an individual's experience of a long night spent in a hospital corridor, although the fact that this may be a rare and atypical incident does not figure in the media's decision to publish. Stories about care in the community tend to focus on cases that have gone disastrously wrong like, for example, people being terrorised by a violent neighbour who has been discharged from an institution. Advertisers also have influence, although this is not direct as they can rarely influence an individual story. However, a newspaper that consistently takes a line that the advertisers disapprove of will lose the advertising revenue that most newspapers depend on to survive.

Who is the audience?

All the media have to be aware of their audience; newspapers especially are aimed at particular groups of people. The *Sun* has a reader demographic that is described as skilled working class, aspiring, right rather than left of centre, with strong views about issues such as asylum seekers, criminals and social security 'scroungers'. The *Daily Mirror* has a very similar audience but retains more of the 'old' Labour voters. The *Guardian* targets the liberal middle class, and the *Daily Mail* targets the traditional middle class. These distinctions may seem absurd, but in relation to newspaper readership they can be supported by demographic profiles, although all newspapers have a minority readership that does not fit the demographic. A paper that strays too far from the views and perceptions of its majority audience will lose circulation and advertisers very quickly.

Is an issue influencing the choice of topic?

When the media discover an issue they decide their readers, viewers or listeners are interested in, they tend also to cover topics relating to the issue such as, for example, current public worries about the increase in obesity, searching them out in preference to other stories. The state of the health and social care services is such an issue, so the media are always interested in topics that illustrate this. However, this can distort the media's coverage of health as other important topics may be neglected as they do not relate to public perception of the issues or, as clearly identified in the King's Fund report *Health in the News*, because the media have misunderstood the real views of the public.

Activity 18.3

Choose a substantial article in a national newspaper and subject it to analysis using these questions.

- Which media (in this case, tabloid or broadsheet)?
- Who owns it (any web search engine will help here; the search question should be, for example, *'Daily Mail* proprietor')?
- What is the quality of the evidence?
- Are commercial pressures influencing the story (the question is always 'who profits')?
- Who is the audience (the search question is, for example, 'reader profile *Daily Mirror*')?
- Is a current issue influencing the choice of topic?

CONCLUSION

This chapter has addressed the topics of how the mass media operates and what the factors influencing the media are. Also, why it is important for health and wellbeing promoters to understand how to interpret and influence the media.

Heightened awareness of the nature of the media can help wellbeing promoters cope with it and use it to their advantage, and also to understand why it is so difficult to get the national media in particular to address positive wellbeing-related messages. It is worth persevering, as active involvement by the public is central to the wellbeing ethos, and an important vehicle for informing and involving the public is the mass media. Wellbeing promoters need to understand media agendas and imperatives and to be actively involved in influencing the media with positive messages about wellbeing.

Further reading and websites

World Health Organization (2009) *Public Health Campaigns: getting the message across* (Mul edition, 27 July 2009)

An interesting and creative approach to using the media to promote health and wellbeing. The WHO has published a compendium of its posters from all over the world.

Hirschhorn, E., Haskins, R. and Nightingale, M. (2008) *Using the Media to Promote Adolescent Wellbeing.* Princeton-Brookings. Available at **http://ccf.tc.columbia.edu/pdf/Children%20and%20Electronic%20 Media_18_01_PolicyBrief.pdf**

This brief advocates the use of media to provide young people with positive messages that counteract the negative and potentially damaging messages to which they are so frequently exposed.

Scottish Government (2003) *Enhancing Sexual Wellbeing in Scotland: a sexual health relationship strategy.* Crown Copyright. Available at **www.scotland.gov.uk/Publications/2003/11/18503/28872** (accessed 15 August 2011)

The Scottish Government shows awareness of the power of the media with regard to health and wellbeing.

Conclusion

Anneyce Knight and Allan McNaught

As this book has identified, concepts of wellbeing have increasingly become an integral part of the policy discourse in modern Britain. There is an established and growing body of literature and research that focuses on different facets of wellbeing, as it concerns individuals, families, communities and societies as a whole. Indeed, the journey of the concept of wellbeing would merit a book of its own. This journey would start with philosophers such as Jeremy Bentham and John Stuart Mill, with their greatest good principle, 'actions are right to the degree that they tend to promote the greatest good for the greatest number'. Today, wellbeing is more frequently associated with 'health' and articulated as subjective wellbeing or happiness. One objective of this book is to place wellbeing in its broader philosophical, social and political context, rather than the softer side of biomedically defined and determined 'health'.

The UK government (2011) intends to collect wellbeing data alongside economic data, following the lead of Bhutan, Canada and France. In trying to explain this interest in developing tools for collecting this data, no one event or work, in the contemporary period, can be pointed to as having propelled wellbeing so far up the political agenda. During the boom years there remained those who pointed to the unfair distribution of economic rewards and that, notwithstanding greater levels of wealth, perceptions of subjective wellbeing, in the West, were not high; thus wealth does not seem to equate directly to wellbeing (Layard, 2005; Wilkinson, 2007).

These conclusions about the link between wealth and wellbeing raised significant questions about the nature of social progress, the role of the state and the distribution of the benefits of economic growth. It is within this context that wellbeing began to be de-linked from its customary coupling with health, and led to its characterisation as a predominantly subjective, psychological construct. The dialect between subjective and objective wellbeing has widened the agenda, raised questions about the nature of wellbeing, and resulted in attempts to reconcile the two levels of meaning. There was no grand plan or design behind this process, but merely scientists following the evidence, and the desire of human beings for progress through individual and societal improvement.

These conceptual developments influenced the context and debates about wellbeing and helped to create a more benign policy climate in which politicians and state agencies joined the discourse, as they saw it to be in their interest to take measures to promote wellbeing. Few, including politicians, could not fail to see benefits in promoting wellbeing as a 'feel-good' concept. This book gives an overview and analysis of facets of both subjective and objective wellbeing. Its overarching argument is that both need to be taken into account as guides to policy and action in modern society. To focus on subjective wellbeing alone individualises responsibility for social, economic and environmental decisions and resource allocation, which the individual is powerless to change, and which are rightly the province of community and political action.

As has been explored in this book, there are many factors involved in attempting to deliver a wellbeing agenda. The challenge for policy makers, practitioners and politicians is to strike a balance between macro and micro elements, and to weigh up the contribution of different social and economic sectors to achieve wellbeing. The Joint Approach to Social Policy (JASP) was an attempt in the 1970s to develop consistent and mutual reinforcing policies, strategies and practices across different areas of social policy. 'Joined-up Government' was the Blairite approach to the same enduring problem.

There is no doubt that the environment and the principles of sustainable development provide one cohesive framework for advancing wellbeing. It is also clear that a partnership and lifespan approach is needed in order to maintain the equilibrium between, for example, environment, design and wellbeing. In addition, the role of education and work in enhancing wellbeing is important. In a time of public sector spending cuts, these areas are increasingly challenged by financial constraints. A wellbeing focus needs to be maintained and extended while we learn how to live within our economic and environmental constraints, as well as within the shifting balance of world economic power.

Individuals do need to know themselves and to be able to access opportunities to develop their wellbeing, whether it is within a spiritual, psychological, social or physical dimension. It is important that all people are seen as individual and that their perception of wellbeing is acknowledged as unique to them. Nevertheless, it is important to recognise that there are societal, cultural and community contexts that influence this perception. This applies equally to the general population and the health, social care and wellbeing professionals who attempt to deliver person-centred care and services.

Those involved in delivering health and social care services, and wellbeing initiatives, will need to increase their awareness of the wide range of tools and resources available in order for 'all' to enhance their wellbeing. Health, social care and wellbeing students and practitioners will also need to be educated to develop innovative and creative ways to meet the challenges ahead to become 'multi-skilled inter sectoral workers'. In addition, understanding the media's influence in promoting wellbeing, and becoming more actively involved in influencing the media with positive messages, will also be necessary as we gain more access to mass media and its representation of wellbeing.

As we have seen, the notion of wellbeing is complex and the sole emphasis cannot be, and should not be, on the individual's subjective feelings. Policy makers, statutory and non-statutory commissioners and service providers have an equal, if not more important, role to play in creating the circumstances that affect our wellbeing. For example, the present (2011) Coalition Government is developing its partnership with food industry representatives in which the latter are taking the lead in committees to develop food policy. Food eaten is an individual choice and affects wellbeing. Individual choice is, however, strongly influenced by those who supply the food, household economics, and media and government campaigns.

Wellbeing is a developing area that should not detract us from the need to address health inequalities, social inclusion and the wider public health agenda. Rather, it should be seen as an integral dimension of twenty-first-century life, and this is exemplified in David Cameron's desire that wellbeing measures should 'steer policy' (Stratton, 2010). However, we would suggest that policy needs to be informed by objective and subjective measures, as well as political commitment to make the changes necessary to enhance wellbeing. *Our Health and Wellbeing Today* (DH, 2010) was issued to accompany the new government's public health White Paper. Within it, the language of wellbeing has been marshalled as a linguistic stance, but the conventional public agenda dominates the document. At the same time, the public health leadership role offered to local authorities, when combined with their wellbeing powers, offers considerable opportunities for innovative work across local government departments, as well as with local partners through LSPs. The new arrangements offer opportunities for innovation and entrepreneurship, despite the constraints of the proposed public expenditure reductions.

The opportunity to develop 'wellbeing' projects is now more of a possibility. It is essential that these projects are robustly monitored and evaluated, both to learn how we can improve our management of complex projects and also to assess the impact on the wellbeing of identified beneficiaries. Without this research and validation of individual project outcomes, it can not be ensured that resources are utilised effectively. This means that health, social care and wellbeing students and practitioners need to be equipped with the necessary skills to manage, monitor and evaluate projects in ways such as detailed project planning, defining evaluation questions, the setting up of indicators, and the setting up of methodological strategies including quantitative and qualitative research methods for collecting data. There are similar needs for community, voluntary and other third sector organisations involved in wellbeing projects, particularly in view of the policy stress on the 'Big Society', localism and the encouragement of social enterprise.

The concept of wellbeing within modern UK society is embryonic. Health, social care and wellbeing students, practitioners and academics need to ensure that it is not a tokenistic term that becomes watered down under the terminology of 'health' or 'happiness', so that 'wellbeing for all' can be achieved.

References

Abbott, R.A., Ploubidis, G.B., Huppert, F.A., Kuh, D., Wadsworth, M.E.J. and Croudance, T.J. (2006) *Health and Quality of Life Outcomes* 4: 76–92

Acheson, D. (1998) *Independent Inquiry into Inequalities in Health*. London: The Stationery Office

Adams, S. (2007) 'Healthy Homes: The Cornerstone of Better Older Age?' Care and Repair England/Warwick 5th Health Housing Conference. Warwick

Ader, R. (2001) 'Psychoneuroimmunology'. *Current Directions in Psychological Science*, 10(3): 94–7

Age Concern (2008) *Housing Policy Position Paper*. Age Concern (2008) as modified in November 2010. Available at: **www.ageuk.org.uk/documents/ en-gb/for-professionals/housing/housing_2008_pro.pdf?dtrk=true** (accessed 15 August 2011)

Ahmad, W.I.U. (1993) *Race and Health in Contemporary Britain*. Buckingham: Open University Press

Ajzen, I. (1991) 'The Theory of Planned Behavior'. *Organizational Behavior and Human Decision Processes*, 50(2): 179–211

Ajzen, I. and Fishbein, M. (1971) 'The production of behavior from attitudinal and normative beliefs'. *Journal of Personality and Social Psychology*, 6: 466–87

Aked, J., Marks, N., Cordon, C. and Thompson, S. (2008) *Five Ways to Wellbeing*. Available at **www.neweconomics.org/sites/neweconomics.org/ files/Five_Ways_to_Well-being_Evidence_1.pdf** (accessed 15 August 2011))

Albrow, R. (1977) *Bureaucracy*. London: Macmillan

Aldous, P. (2010) 'Neighbourhoods that can kill'. *New Scientist*, 2743: 6–9

Alford, R. (1975) *Health Care Politics: ideological and interest group barriers to reform*. Chicago: Chicago University Press

Allan, S. and Gilbert, P. (2002) 'Anger and anger expression in relation to perceptions of social rank, entrapment and depressive symptoms'. *Personality and Individual Differences*, 551–65

Allan, T. (2005) 'Private sector housing improvement in the UK and the chronically ill: implications for collaborative working'. *Housing Studies*, 20(1): 63–80

Allardt, E. (1976) 'Dimensions of welfare in a comparative Scandinavian study'. *Acta Sociologica*, 19 (227–40), in Konu, A. and Rimpelä, M. (2002) 'Well-being in schools: a conceptual model'. *Health Promotion International*, 17(1): 79–87

AMOSSHE (2009) *The Association of Managers of Student Services in Higher Education Supplement to the HEFCE financial sustainability strategy group (FSSG) report: The sustainability of learning and teaching in English higher education.* Available at **www.amosshe.org.uk/amosshe/assets/_managed/editor/FSSG%20supplement.pdf** (accessed 15 August 2011)

Andersson, J., Libby, P. and Hansson, G.K. (2010) 'Adaptive immunity and atherosclerosis'. *Clinical Immunology*, 134(1): 33–46

Andoh, A., Ogawa, A., Bamba, S. and Fujiyam, Y. (2007) 'Interaction between interleukin-17-producing CD4+ T cells and colonic subepithelial myofibroblasts: what are they doing in mucosal inflammation?' *Journal of Gastroenterology*, 17(42): 29–33

Andreu, A.L., Hanna, M.G., Reichmann, H., Bruno, C., Penn, A.S., Tanji, K., Allotti, F., Iwata, S., Bonilla, E., Lach, B., Morgan-Hughes, J. and DiMauro, S. (1999) 'Exercise intolerance due to mutations in the cytochrome *b* gene of mitochondrial DNA'. *New England Journal of Medicine*, 341: 1037–44

Antonovsky, A. (1979) *Health, Stress and Coping.* San Francisco: Jossey-Bass

Ardell, D.B. (1985) 'The history and future of wellness'. *Health Values*, 9(6): 37–56

Aristotle (1985) *Nichomachean Ethics* (T. Irwin, translator). Indianapolis: Hackett Publishing Company

Aronson, E., Wilson, T. and Akert, R. (2005) *Social Psychology* (5th Ed). London: Houghton Mifflin

Arts Council England (2005) *Arts, Creativity and Health in the South East.* Brighton: Arts Council England

Aubert, G. and Lansdorp, P.M. (2008) 'Telomeres and Aging'. *Physiological Reviews*, 88(2): 557–79

Audit Commission (2009) *Building Better Lives: getting the best from strategic housing.* London: Audit Commission

Auletta, K. (1982) *The Underclass.* New York: Random House

Australian National Bureau of Statistics (2002) *Discussion paper: social capital and social wellbeing.* Canberra: Australian National Bureau of Statistics

Baer, R.A., Smith, G.T. and Allen, K.B. (2004) 'Assessment of mindfulness by self-report. The Kentucky inventory of mindfulness skills'. *Assessment*, 11: 191–206

Bakrhe, M.S. and Morgan, W.P. (1978) 'Anxiety reduction following exercise and meditation'. *Cognitive Therapy and Research*, 2: 323–33

Bakshi, R. (2007) *An Economics for Well-being.* Mumbai: Centre for Education and Documentation

Bambra, C., Fox, D. and Scott-Samuel, A. (2003) 'Towards a new politics of health' Discussion Paper 1. Liverpool: Politics of Health Group

Bandura, A. (1977) 'Self-efficacy: toward a unifying theory of behavioral change'. *Psychological Review*, 84: 191–215

Barker, R. (ed) (2009) *Making Sense of Every Child Matters: Multi-professional practice guidance.* London: Policy Press

Barnes, J., Belsky, J., Broomfield, K.A., Dave, S., Frost, M. and Melhuish, E. (2005) 'Disadvantaged but different: variation among deprived communities in relation to child and family wellbeing. The National Evaluation of Sure Start Research Team'. *Journal of Child Psychology and Psychiatry*, 46(9): 952–62. In Wollny *et al.* (2010)

Barry, A.M. and Yuill, C. (2008) *Understanding the Sociology of Health* (2nd Ed). London: Sage Publications

Bartholomew, J.B. and Linder, D.E. (1998) 'State anxiety following resistance exercise: the role of gender and exercise intensity'. *Journal of Behavioral Medicine*, 21: 205–19

Bauer, J.J. and McAdams, D.P. (2004) 'Growth goals, maturity, and well-being'. *Developmental Psychology*, 40: 114–27

BBC Radio Nottingham (2001) *Writing a Press Release with IMPACT.* Available at **www.bbc.co.uk/nottingham/community/presser.shtml** (accessed 15 August 2011)

Beattie, A., Gott, M., Jones, L. and Sidell, M. (1993) *Health and Well-being: a reader:* Basingstoke: Macmillan and Open University Press

Beauchamp, T. and Childress, J. (2001) *Principle of Biomedical Ethics* (5th Ed). Oxford: Oxford University Press

Bennett, M.P., Zeller, J.M., Rosenberg, L. and McCann, J. (2003) 'The effect of mirthful laughter on stress and natural killer cell activity'. *Alternative Therapy and Health Medicine*, 9(2): 38–45

Bentham, J. (1780) *An Introduction to the Principles of Morals and Legislation.* Chapter 1: 'Of the Principle of Utility'. Available at **http://oll.libertyfund. org/index.php?option=com_staticxt&staticfile=show.php%3Ftitle=192 0&Itemid=99999999** (accessed 15 August 2011)

Bentham, J. (1817) 'Chrestomathia', in *The Works of Jeremy Bentham*, vol. 8 *(Chrestomathia, Essays on Logic and Grammar, Tracts on Poor Laws, Tracts on Spanish Affairs)* (p.79). Online. Available at **http://oll.libertyfund. org/index.php?option=com_staticxt&staticfile=show.php%3Ftitle=192 0&Itemid=99999999** (accessed 15 August 2011)

Bentham, J. (1969) 'An introduction to the principles of morals and legislation', cited in Hart H.L.A. and Burns, J.H. (1996) *The Collected Works of Jeremy Bentham: An introduction to the principles of morals and legislation*. Oxford: Clarendon Press

Benyamini, Y., Leventhal, E.A. and Leventhal, H. (2000) 'Gender differences in processing information for making self-assessments of health'. *Psychosomatic Medicine*, 62: 354–64

Berger, B.G. (2004) 'Subjective well-being in obese individuals: the multiple roles of exercise'. *Quest*, 56(1): 50–76

Biddle, S.J.H., Fox, K.R. and Boutcher, S.H. (2000) *Physical Activity and Psychological Well being.* London: Routledge

Bioregional (2010) *Beddington Zero Energy Development* (BedZED). Available at **www.bioregional.com** (accessed 15 August 2011)

Black, C. (2008) *Dame Carol Black's Review of the health of Britain's working-age population 'Working for a healthier tomorrow'*, 17 March 2008. London: TSO. Available at **www.dwp.gov.uk/docs/hwwb-working-for-a-healthier-tomorrow.pdf** (accessed 15 August 2011)

Blanchflower, D.G. and Oswald, A.J. (2004) 'Wellbeing over time in Britain and the USA'. *Journal of Public Economics*, 88:1359–86

Blanchflower, D.G. and Oswald, A.J. (2008) 'Is well-being U-shaped over the life cycle?' *Social Science & Medicine*, 66(8): 1733–49

Bluhm, G., Nordling, E. and Berglind, N. (2004) 'Road traffic noise and annoyance – an increasing environmental health problem'. *Noise and Health*, 6(24): 43–9

Blumenthal, J.A., Babyak, M.A., Moore, K.A., Craighead, W.E., Herman, S., Khatri, P., Waugh, R., Napolitano, M.A., Forman, L.M., Appelbaum, M., Doraiswamy, P.M. and Krishnan, K.R. (1999) 'Effects of exercise training on older patients with major depression'. *Archives of Internal Medicine*, 159: 2349–56

Bond, E.J. (1996) *Ethics and Human Well Being: an introduction to moral philosophy*. London: Blackwell Publishers

Bonomi, A.E., Boudreau, D.M., Fishman, P.A., Meenan, R.T. and Revicki, D.A. (2005) 'Is a family equal to the sum of its parts? Estimating family-level well-being for cost-effectiveness analysis'. *Quality of Life Research*, 14: 1127–33.

Bonvallet, M. and Bloch, V. (1961) 'Bulbar control of cortical arousal'. *Science*, 133:1133–4

Bottomore, T. (1970) *Elites and Society*. Harmondsworth: Pelican

Bourne, P.A. (2010) 'A conceptual framework of wellbeing in some Western nations'. *Current Research Journal of Social Sciences*, 2(1): 15–23

Boutcher, S.H. (1999) 'Cognitive performance, fitness and ageing', in Biddle, S.J.H., Fox, K.R. and Boutcher, S.H. (eds) *Physical Activity and Psychological Well-being*. London: Routledge

Briner, R. and Dewberry, C. (2007) Staff Wellbeing is Key to School Success. Available at **www.worklifesupport.com/with/education/?assetdetesc tl62948=250** (accessed 15 August 2011)

British Trust for Conservation Volunteers (BTCV) (2009) *Investing in Sustainable Futures: BTCV Strategic Plan 2009–2013*. Available at **www2. btcv.org.uk/btcv_strategy_09-13.pdf** (accessed 15 August 2011)

British Trust for Conservation Volunteers (BTCV) (2010) *Green Gym Camden*. Available at **www2.btcv.org.uk/display/btcv_ggcamden** (accessed 15 August 2011)

Brown, K.W. and Ryan, R.M. (2003) 'The benefits of being present: mindfulness and its role in psychological well-being'. *Journal of Personality and Social Psychology*, 84: 822–48

Bruneau, B.M.S. (2009) *A Study of the Association Between Undergraduates' Resilience and their Coping*. Unpublished thesis: University of Wales

Bryant, P.A., Trinder, J. and Curtis, N. (2004) 'Sick and tired: does sleep have a vital role in the immune system?' *Nature Reviews Immunology*, 4: 457–67

Buchanan, D.R. (2000) *An Ethics for Health Promotion Rethinking the Sources of Human Well Being*. Oxford: Oxford University Press

Buckley, T.M. and Schatzberg, A.F. (2005) 'On the interactions of the Hypothalamic-Pituitary-Adrenal (HPA) axis and sleep: normal HPA axis activity and circadian rhythm, exemplary sleep disorders'. *The Journal of Clinical Endocrinology & Metabolism*, 90(5): 3106–14

Buckworth, J. and Dishman, R.K. (2002) *Exercise Psychology*. Champaign, IL: Human Kinetics

Building Research Establishment (BRE) and Chartered Institute of Environmental Health (CIEH) (2008) *Good Housing Leads to Good Health: a toolkit for environmental health practitioners*. London: CIEH

Calfas, K.J. and Taylor, W.C. (1994) 'Effects of physical activity on psychological variables in adolescents'. *Pediatric Exercise Science*, 6: 402–23

Callinicos, A.T. (2003) *The New Mandarins of American Power*. Cambridge: Polity Press

Cameron, E., Mathers, J. and Parry, J. (2006) 'Health and wellbeing: questioning the use of health concepts in public health policy and practice'. *Critical Public Health*, 16(4): 347–54

Camfield, L., Streuli, N. and Woodhead, M. (2008) *What's the use of 'wellbeing' in contexts of child poverty? Approaches to research, monitoring and children's participation*. Oxford: University of Oxford

Camfield, L. and Skevington, S.M. (2008) 'On subjective well-being and quality of life'. *Health Psychology*, 13(6): 764–75

Campbell, D.W., Sareen, J., Stein, M.B., Kravetsky, L.B., Paulus, M.P., Hassard, S.T. and Reiss, J.P. (2009) Happy but not so approachable: the social judgements of individuals with generalized social phobia. *Depression and Anxiety*, 26(5): 419–24

Canli, T. and Lesch, K. (2007) 'Long story short: the serotonin transporter in emotion regulation and social cognition'. *Nature Neuroscience*, 10: 1103–9

Carland-Adams, B. (2010) 'Educational achievement improved by national school lunch program'. *Medical News Today*. Available at **www.medicalnewstoday.com/articles/192510.php** (accessed 15 August 2011)

Carlson, R.J. (1975) *The End of Medicine*. New York: Wiley

Cattan, M., White, M., Bond, J. and Learmouth, A. (2005) 'Preventing social isolation and loneliness among older people: a systematic review of health promotion interventions'. *Ageing & Society*, 25: 41–67

Cattrell, V. and Herring, R. (2002) 'Social capital, generations and health in East London', in Swann, C. and Morgan, A. (eds) *Social Capital: insights from qualitative research*. London: Health Development Agency

Cavill, N. (ed) (2007) *Building Health: blueprint for action*. London: National Heart Forum

CDC-US Department of Health and Human Services (1996) *Physical Activity and Health: a report of the Surgeon General*. US Department of Health and Human Services, Centers for Disease Control and Prevention. Atlanta, GA: National Center for Chronic Disease Prevention and Health Promotion

Chapman, L. and West-Burnham, J. (2010) *Education for Social Justice*. London: Continuum

Chartered Institute of Environmental Health (2010) *Annual Survey of Noise Enforcement – Results for 2008–09*. Available at: **www.cieh.org/uploadedFiles/Core/Policy/Environmental_protection/Noise/UK_noise_results_2008-9.pdf** (accessed 15 August 2011)

Chauloff, F. (1997) 'The serotonin hypothesis'. In: *Physical activity and mental health*, Morgan, W.P. (ed). Washington, DC: Taylor & Francis, pp. 179–198

Checkland, K. (2004) 'National Service Frameworks and UK general practitioners: street-level bureaucrats at work?'. *Sociology of Health and Illness*, 26(7): 951–71

Cheminais, R. (2008) *How to Achieve the Every Child Matters Standards: a practical guide*. London: Sage

Cheminais, R. (2009) *Effective Multi-Agency Partnerships: putting Every Child Matters into practice*. London: Sage

Cheng, S.T. and Chang, A.C.M. (2005) 'Measuring psychological well-being in the Chinese'. *Personality & Individual Differences*, 38(6): 1307–16

Cherry, A. and Hodkinson, R. (2009) 'Millennium Homes Revisited'. *Ingenia*, 41: 39–44

City of Westminster (2010) *Westminster Noise Strategy 2010–2015*. Available at http://westminster.gov.uk/workspace/assets/publications/Final-Westminster-Noise-Strategy-1269269299.pdf (accessed 15 August 2011)

Cockerham, W.C. (2007) *Medical Sociology* (10th Ed). New Jersey: Pearson, Prentice-Hall

Cohen, D., McKenzie, T., Sehgal, A., Williamson, S., Golinelli, D. and Lurie, N. (2007) 'Contribution of Public Parks to Physical Activity'. *American Journal of Public Health*, 97(3): 509–14

Colberg, S.R., Somma, C.T. and Sechrist, S.R. (2008) 'Physical activity participation may offset some of the negative impact of diabetes on cognitive function'. *Journal of the American Medical Directors' Association*, 9(6): 434–8

Commission for Architecture and the Built Environment (CABE) (2009) *Future Health: sustainable places for health and wellbeing*. London: CABE. Also online at http://webarchive.nationalarchives.gov.uk/20110118095356/http:/www.cabe.org.uk/files/future-health.pdf (accessed 15 August 2011)

Committee of Public Accounts (2002) *Tackling obesity in England*. Available at www.publications.parliament.uk/pa/cm200102/cmselect/cmpubacc/421/42103.htm (accessed 15 August 2011)

Conrad, P. (1994) 'Wellness as a virtue: morality and the pursuit of health'. *Culture, Medicine and Psychiatry*, 18(3): 385–401

Craft, L.L. and Landers, D.M. (1998) 'The effect of exercise on clinical depression and depression resulting from mental illness: a meta-analysis'. *Journal of Sports and Exercise Psychology*, 20: 339–57

Crisp, R. (2003) *How Should One Live?* Oxford: Oxford University Press

Crisp, R. (2008) 'Well Being', in *Stanford Encyclopaedia of Philosophy*. Available at http://plato.stanford.edu/entries/well-being/ (accessed 15 August 2011)

Cronin de Chavez, A., Backett-Milburn, K., Parry, O. and Platt, S. (2005) 'Understanding and researching wellbeing: its usage in different disciplines and potential for health research and health promotion'. *Health Education Journal*, 64(1): 70–87

Croucher, K., Hicks, L. and Jackson, K. (2006) *Housing with Care for Later Life: a literature review*. York: Joseph Rowntree Foundation

Croucher, K., Myers, L. and Bretherton, J. (2008) *The links between greenspace and health: a critical literature review.* Greenspace Scotland. Available at **www.greenspacescotland.org.uk/upload/File/the%20links%20between%20greenspace%20and%20health%20critical%20literature%20review%20Oct07.pdf** (accessed 15 August 2011)

Crow, F. (2008) 'A well-being imperative: empowering schools, improving outcomes'. A presentation given to the East Sussex County Council Inclusive Learning team, 10 December 2008

Culliford, L. (2009) 'Teaching spirituality and health care to third-year medical students'. *Clinical Teacher,* 6(1): 22–7

Dahl, R. (1957) 'The concept of power', in Clark, T. (1968) *Community Structure and Decision-making.* Scranton, PA: Chandler

Dahl, R. (1961) *Who Governs?* New Haven, CT: Yale University Press

Damasio, A.R. (2000) 'A second chance for emotion' (Chapter 2, pp. 12–23), in Lane, R.D. and Nadel, L. (eds) *Cognitive Neuroscience of Emotion.* Oxford: Oxford University Press

Danna, K. and Griffin, R.W. (1999) 'Health and wellbeing in the workplace: a review and synthesis of the literature'. *Journal of Management,* 25(3): 357–84

Daruna, J.H. (2004) *Introduction to Psychoneuroimmunology.* London: Elsevier

Darwin, C. (2007) *The Expression of the Emotions in Man and Animals.* Minneapolis, MN: Filiquarian Publishing, LLC

Davidson, M., Roys, M., Nicol, S., Ormandy, D. and Ambrose, P. (2009) *The Real Cost of Poor Housing.* Bracknell: IHS BRE Press

Davis, S., Porteus, J. and Skidmore, C. (2009) *Housing, Health and Care.* Coventry: CIH and Housing Learning and Improvement Network

DeBrabander, B. and Gerits, P. (1999) 'Chronic and acute stress as predictors of relapse in primary breast cancer patients'. *Patient Education and Counselling,* 37: 265–72

Deci, E.L. and Ryan, R.R. (2008) 'Hedonia, eudaimonia, and well being: an introduction'. *Journal of Happiness Studies,* 9: 1–11

Delahanty, L.M., Meigs, J.B., Hayden, D., Williamson, D.A. and Nathan, D.M. (2002) Diabetes Prevention Program (DPP) Research Group. 'Psychological and behavioral correlates of baseline BMI in the diabetes prevention program (DPP)'. *Diabetes Care,* 25(11):1992–8

De Leon, E. and Boris, E. (2010) *The State of Society: measuring economic success and human well-being.* Washington, DC: Urban Institute

Department for Environment, Food and Rural Affairs (DEFRA) (2006) *Securing the Future: UK government sustainable development strategy.* London: DEFRA

Department for Environment, Food and Rural Affairs (DEFRA) (2008) *Outdoors for All? An Action Plan to increase the number of people from under-represented groups who access the natural environment.* Available at: **http://archive.defra.gov.uk/rural/documents/countryside/dap-ofa.pdf** (accessed 15 August 2011)

Department for Environment, Food and Rural Affairs (DEFRA) (2009) *Sustainable development indicators in your pocket.* London: DEFRA

Department for Environment, Food and Rural Affairs (DEFRA) (2010a) *Measuring Progress: sustainable development indicators* 2010. Available at http://sd.defra.gov.uk/documents/SDI2010_001.pdf (accessed 15 August 2011)

Department for Environment, Food and Rural Affairs (DEFRA) (2010b) *Noise Policy Statement for England.* Available at http://archive.defra.gov.uk/environment/quality/noise/policy/documents/noise-policy.pdf (accessed 15 August 2011)

Department of Children, Schools and Families (DCSF) (2005) *Every Child Matters*

Department of Communities and Local Government (DCLG) (2006) *Strong and Prosperous Communities: the local government white paper.* Available at www.communities.gov.uk/strongprosperouscommunitieswp (accessed 15 August 2011)

Department of Communities and Local Government (DCLG) (2007) *Place Matters.* Available at http://www.communities.gov.uk/documents/communities/pdf/153370.pdf (accessed 15 August 2011)

Department of Communities and Local Government (DCLG) (2009) *World Class Places: the government's strategy for improving quality of place.* Available at www.communities.gov.uk/publications/communities/worldclassplaces (accessed 15 August 2011)

Department of Communities and local Government (DCLG) (2009) *Power to promote well-being of the area: Statutory guidance for local councils.* London: DCLG

Department of Health (DH) (2007) *Guidance on Joint Strategic Needs Assessment.* London: DH

Department of Health (DH) (2009) *Flourishing People, Connected Communities. A framework for developing well-being.* London: DH

Department of Health (DH) (2009a) *NHS Health and Wellbeing Review: interim report* London: DH

Department of Health (DH) (2009b) *Health and Wellbeing Assessment: questions and guidance for regulatory impact assessment.* Available at www.dh.gov.uk/en/Publicationsandstatistics/Legislation/Healthassessment/DH_4093626 (accessed 15 August 2011)

Department of Health (DH) (2010) *Key Vaccine Information: MMR.* Available at http://www.dh.gov.uk/en/Publichealth/Immunisation/Keyvaccineinformation/DH_103952 (accessed 15 August 2011)

Department of Health (DH) (2010) *Equity and Excellence: liberating the NHS.* The Stationery Office Ltd. Available at www.dh.gov.uk/en/Publicationsandstatistics/Publications/PublicationsPolicyAndGuidance/DH_117353 (accessed 15 August 2011)

Department of Health (DH) (2010) *Our Health and Wellbeing Today.* London: DH

Department of Health Chief Medical Officer (2002) *On the State of Public Health.* Available at www.dh.gov.uk/prod_consum_dh/groups/dh_digitalassets/@dh/@en/documents/digitalasset/dh_4081860.pdf (accessed 15 August 2011)

Department of Health (DH), Department for Work and Pensions (DWP) and the Health and Safety Executive (HSE) (2005) Health, Work and Wellbeing:

caring for our future. A strategy for the health and wellbeing of working-age people. Available at www.dh.gov.uk/en/Publicationsandstatistics/Publications/PublicationsPolicyAndGuidance/DH_4121756 (accessed 15 August 2011)

Department for Work and Pensions (DWP) and Department of Health (DH) (2008) Improving Health and Work: changing lives. Available at www.dwp.gov.uk/docs/hwwb-improving-health-and-work-changing-lives.pdf (accessed 15 August 2011)

Depledge, M. and Bird, W. (2009) 'The Blue Gym: health and wellbeing from our coasts'. *Marine Pollution Bulletin*, 58: 947–8

Design Council (2009) *Villiers High School*. Available at www.designcouncil.org.uk/case-studies/design-out-crime/villiers-high-school/ (accessed 15 August 2011)

Diabetes Prevention Program Research Group (DPP) (2002) 'Reduction in the incidence of type 2 diabetes with lifestyle intervention or metformin'. *New England Journal of Medicine*, 346: 393–403

Didonna, F. (2009) *Mindfulness-Based Approaches to Eating Disorders*. New York: Springer

Diener, E. (1984) 'Subjective well being'. *Psychological Bulletin*, 95: 542–75

Diener, E. (2005) *Guidelines for National Indicators of Subjective Well-Being and Ill-Being*, Chicago: University of Illinois

Diener, E. (2009) *The Science of Wellbeing: the collected works of Ed Diener*. New York: Springer Dordrecht

Diener, E. and Biswas-Diener, R. (2002) 'Will money increase subjective well-being?'. *Social Indicator Research*, 57:119–69

Diener, E. and Diener, E. (1995) 'Cross-cultural correlates of life satisfaction and self-esteem'. *Journal of Personality and Social Psychology* 68(4): 653–63

Diener, E., Lucas, E.L. and Oishi, S. (2002) 'Subjective well-being', in Snyder, C.R. and Lopez, S.J. (eds) *Handbook of Positive Psychology* (Chapter 3, pp. 63–73). New York: Oxford University Press

Diener, E., Lucas, R.L. and Scollon, C.N. (2009) 'Beyond the hedonic treadmill'. *Revising the Adaptation Theory of Well-Being*, 37. Netherlands: Springer

Diener, E., Oishi, S. and Lucas, R.E. (2003) 'Personality, culture, and subjective well-being: emotional and cognitive evaluations of life'. *Annual Review of Psychology*, 54: 403–25

Diener, E. and Seligman, M.E. (2002).'Very happy people'. *Psychology Science*, 13(1): 81–4

Diener, E. and Seligman, E. (2004) 'Beyond Money: towards an economy of wellbeing?' *Psychological Science in the Public Interest*, 5(1): 1–31

Dierich, M. (2007) 'Adventures in health care: designing a wellness center for low-income elders'. *Urologic Nursing*, 27(5): 403–8

Di Loreto, C., Fanelli, C., Lucidi, P., Murdolo, G., De Cicco, A., Parlanti, N., Ranchelli, A., Fatone, C., Taglioni, C., Santeusanio, F. and De Feo, P. (2005) 'Make your diabetic patients walk: long-term impact of different amounts of physical activity on type 2 diabetes'. *Diabetes Care*, 28(6): 1295–302

Dishman, R.K. (1997) 'The norepinefrine hypothesis' (pp. 199–212), in Morgan, W.P. (ed) *Physical Activity and Mental Health*. Washington, DC: Taylor & Francis

Doak, S. and Kusel, J. (1996) 'Well-being in forest dependent communities, Part II: A social assessment focus', in *Sierra-Nevada Ecosystem Project: Final Report to Congress, Vol. II, Assessments and scientific basis for management options, University of California, Centers for Water and Wildland Resources*. California: Davis

Dolan, P., Peasgood, T., Dixon, A., Knight, M., Phillips, D., Tsuchiya, A. and White, A. (2006) *Research on the relationship between well-being and sustainable development*. London: DEFRA

Doll, R. (1992) 'Health and empowerment in the 1990s'. *American Journal of Public Health*, 82: 933–41

Donald, I.P. (2009) 'Housing and health care for older people'. *Age and Ageing*, 38(4): 346–67

Donovan, J. (1984) 'Ethnicity and health: a research review'. *Social Science and Medicine*, 19(7): 663–70

Dubos, R. (1959) 'Utopias and Human Goals.' *Mirage of Health: utopias, progress and biological change*. New York: Harper & Brothers Publishers

Dugmore, L., Tipson, R., Phillips, M., Flint, E., Stentiford, N., Bone, M. and Littler, W. (1999) 'Changes in cardiorespiratory fitness, psychological wellbeing, quality of life, and vocational status following a 12-month cardiac exercise rehabilitation programme'. *Heart*, 81(4): 359–66

Duncan, R. (2000) *Globalisation and Income Inequality. An International Perspective*. Given at the 5th Annual Conference on International Trade Education and Research. Melbourne, 26–27 October 2000

Earl, S., Carden, F. and Smutylo, T. (2001) *Outcome Mapping: building learning and reflection into development programmes*, IDRC. Available at www.idrc.ca/openebooks/959-3/ (accessed 15 August 2011)

Eastern Region Public Health Observatory (2005) *Monitoring Childhood Obesity: an update*. Available at www.erpho.org.uk/Download/Public/12598/1/04%20Monitoring%20child%20obesity%20on%20A4%20final.pdf (accessed 15 August 2011)

Economic and Social Research Council (ESRC) (2010) Census questions, forms and definitions. Available at www.census.ac.uk/guides/Qf.aspx (accessed 15 August 2011)

Eid, M. and Diener, E. (2001) 'Norms for experiencing emotions in different cultures: inter- and intra-national differences'. *Journal of Personality and Social Psychology*, 81(5): 869–85

Elenkov, I.J., Iezzoni, D.G., Daly, A., Harris, A.G. and Chrousos, G.P. (2005) 'Cytokine dysregulation, inflammation and well-being'. *Neuroimmunomodulation*, 12(5): 255–69

Elmore, R. (1979) 'Backward mapping: implementation research and policy decision'. *Policy Sciences Quarterly*, 94(4): 601–16

Ereaut, G. and Wright, R. (2008) *What do we mean by 'wellbeing'? And why might it matter?* Research Report DCSF-RW073. London: DCSF

Etnier, J.L., Salazar, W., Landers D.M., Petruzzello, S.J., Han, M. and Nowell,

P. (1997) 'The influence of physical fitness and exercise upon cognitive functioning: a meta-analysis'. *Journal of Sport and Exercise Psychology*, 19: 249–74

European Commission (2004) *Joint Report on Social Exclusion*. Available at http://ec.europa.eu/employment_social/soc-prot/soc-incl/final_joint_inclusion_report_2003_en.pdf (accessed 15 August 2011)

European Commission (2008) Brussels *European Union Physical Activity Guidelines*

European Environment Agency (2010) *Environmental Terminology and Discovery Service*. Available at http://glossary.eea.europa.eu/terminology/concept_html?term=environmental%20quality (accessed 15 August 2011)

Evans, D. (2004) 'Shifting the balance of power? UK public health policy and capacity building'. *Critical Public Health*, 14(1): 63–75

Evans, G. (2005) 'Measure for measure: evaluating the evidence of culture's contribution to regeneration'. *Urban Studies*, 42(5/6): 959–83

Express India (2009) 'Wellness market to grow by 30–35% in 5 years'. New Delhi, *Express India*, 15 April. Available at www.expressindia.com/latest-news/Wellness-market-to-grow-at-3035-pc-in-5-yrs/447267/ (accessed 15 August 2011)

Faculty of Public Health (2010) *Great Outdoors: how our natural health service uses green space to improve wellbeing. An action report*. Available at www.fph.org.uk/uploads/r_great_outdoors.pdf (accessed 15 August 2011)

Farooqi, S., Rau, H., Whitehead, J. and O'Rahilly. S. (1998) '*ob* gene mutations and human obesity'. *Proceedings of the Nutrition Society*, 57: 471–5

Faulkner, G. and Taylor, A.H. (2005) *Exercise, Health and Mental Health: emerging relationships*. London: Routledge

Fava, G.A., Ruini, C., Rafanelli, C., Finos, L., Salmaso, L., Mangelli, L., et al. (2003) 'Well-being therapy of generalized anxiety disorder'. *Psychotherapy and Psychosomatics*, 74(1): 26–30

Felce, D. and Perry, J. (1995) 'Quality of life; its definition and measurement'. *Research in Developmental Disabilities*, 16(1): 51–4

Feldman, F. (2004) *Pleasure and the Good Life*. Gloucestershire: Clarendon Press

Ferrarini, R., Carbognin, C., Casarotti, E.M., Nicolis, E., Nencini, A. and Meneghini, A.M. (2010) 'The emotional response to wine consumption'. *Food Quality and Preference*, 21: 720–5. Available at www.sciencedirect.com/science?_ob=MImg&_imagekey=B6T6T-50BJNKB-2-3&_cdi=5039&_user=6850876&_pii=S095032931000114X&_origin=search&_zone=rslt_list_item&_coverDate=10%2F31%2F2010&_sk=999789992&wchp=dGLbVlW-zSkWb&md5=eefad553ac6032bff79ac27e36d69c11&ie=/sdarticle.pdf (accessed 15 August 2011)

Finlayson, G., King, N. and Blundell, J.E. (1999) 'Liking vs. wanting food: importance for human appetite control and weight regulation'. *Neuroscience & Biobehavioural Reviews*, 31(7): 987–1002

Fishbein, M. and Ajzen, I. (1975) *Belief, Attitude, Intention, and Behavior: an introduction to theory and research*. Reading, MA: Addison-Wesley

Fisher, J., Francis, L. and Johnson, P. (2000) 'Assessing spiritual health via four domains of spiritual wellbeing: the SH4DI'. *Pastoral Psychology*, 49(2):133–45

Fitzgerald, F.T. (1994) 'The tyranny of health'. *New England Journal of Medicine*, 331(3):196–8

Flateau, P., Galea, J. and Petridis, R. (2000) 'Mental health & wellbeing and employment'. *Australian Economic Review*, 3,(2):161–81

Foley, M. (2010) *The Age of Absurdity*. London: Simon and Schuster UK Ltd

Food Climate Research Network (2008) *Cooking up a storm: food greenhouse gas emissions and our climate change*. Available at **www.fcrn.org.uk/sites/default/files/CuaS_web.pdf** (accessed 15 August 2011)

Food Standards Agency (FSA) (2004) *Food Standards Agency Strategic Plan 2005–2010: putting consumers first*. Available at **www.food.gov.uk/multimedia/pdfs/stratplan0510.pdf** (accessed 15 August 2011)

Food Standards Agency (FSA) (2009) *Tips on Chips: help businesses serve healthier food*. Available at **www.food.gov.uk/multimedia/pdfs/chipadvice.pdf** (accessed 15 August 2011)

Food Standards Agency (FSA) (2010) *Agency publishes salt commitments*, 25 March 2010. Available at **www.food.gov.uk/news/newsarchive/2010/mar/saltcommitments** (accessed 15 August 2011)

Food Vision (2009) *Gateshead Salt Shaker Project*. Available at **www.foodvision.gov.uk/pages/gateshead-salt-shaker-study** (accessed 15 August 2011)

Foresight (2008) *Mental Capital and Wellbeing*. Available at **www.foresight.gov.uk/Mental%20Capital/Mental_capital_&_wellbeing_Exec_Sum.pdf** (accessed 15 August 2011)

Foucault, M. (1973) *The Birth of the Clinic*. London: Tavistock

Fox, K.R. (1999) 'The influence of physical activity on mental well-being'. *Public Health Nutrition*, 2: 411–18

Fox, K.R. (2000a) 'Self-esteem, self-perceptions and exercise'. *International Journal of Sports Psychology*, 31: 228–40

Fox, K.R. (2000b) 'The influence of exercise on self-perceptions and self-esteem' (pp. 88–111), in Biddle, S.J.H., Fox K.R. and Boutcher S.H. (eds) *Physical Activity and Psychological Well-being*. London: Routledge

Francis, G., Bishop, L., Luke, C., Middleton, B., Williams, P. and Arendt, J. (2008) 'Sleep during the Antarctic winter: preliminary observations on changing the spectral composition of artificial light'. *Journal of Sleep Research*, 17: 354–60.

Friedman, M. and Friedman, R. (1980) *Free to Choose: a personal statement*. New York: Harcourt Brace Jovanovich

Froy, F. and Giguère, S. (2008) 'Breaking out of silos: joining up policy locally'. A working paper by the OECD Local Economic and Employment Development Programme. Paris: OECD

Gallie, W.C.B. (1956) 'Essentially contested concepts'. *Proceedings of the Aristotelian Society*, 56: 67–198

Ganesh, S. and McAllum, K. (2010) 'Well-being as discourse: potentials and problems for studies of organizing and health inequalities'. *Management Communication Quarterly*, 24(3): 491–8

Gans, H.J. (1995) *The War Against the Poor: the underclass, anti-poverty policy.* New York: Basic Books

Gardiner, P. (2003) 'A virtue ethics approach to moral dilemmas in medicine'. *Journal of Medical Ethics*, 29(5): 297–302

Gardner, H. (1983) *Frames of Mind: The theory of multiple intelligences.* New York: Basic Books

George, M.S., Ketter, T.A., Parekh, P.I., Herscovitch, P. and Post, R.M. (1996) 'Gender differences in regional cerebral blood flow during transient self-induced sadness or happiness'. *Biological Psychiatry*, 40(9):859–71

Giddens, A. (1989) *Sociology*, Cambridge: Polity Press

Gidlöf-Gunnarsson, A. and Öhrström, E. (2007) 'Noise and wellbeing in urban residential environments: the potential role of perceived availability and nearby green areas'. *Landscape and Urban Planning*, 83(2–3):115–26

Gilbert, P. (2008) 'The relationship of shame, social anxiety and depression: the role of the evaluation of social rank'. *Clinical Psychology & Psychotherapy*, 7(3): 174–89

Glover, D.A., Steele, A.C., Stuber, M.L. and Fahey, J.L. (2005) 'Preliminary evidence for lymphocyte distribution differences at rest and after acute psychological stress in PTSD-symptomatic women'. *Brain Behaviour and Immunity*, 19: 243–51

Goldney, R.D., Phillips, P.J., Fisher, L.J. and Wilson D.H. (2004) 'Diabetes, depression, and quality of life: a population study'. *Diabetes Care*, 27: 1066–70

Goldsby, R.A., Kindt, T.J. and Osborne, B.A. (2002) *Immunology* (4th Ed). New York: Freeman and Company

Golonzhka, O., Leid, M., Indra, G. and Indra, A.K. (2007) 'Expression of COUP-TF-interacting protein 2 (CTIP2) in mouse skin during development and in adulthood'. *Gene Expression Patterns*, 7(7): 754–60

Grace, C. and Whiteman, R. (2010) 'Public service futures', in Tuddenham, R. (ed) *The big society: next practice and public service futures.* London: The Guardian-Public

Groenewegen, P., van den Berg, A., de Vries, S. and Verheij, R. (2006) 'Vitamin G: effects of green space on health, well-being, and social safety'. *BMC Public Health*, 6:149. Available at **www.biomedcentral.com/1471-2458/6/149** (accessed 15 August 2011)

Groenvold, M., Petersen, M.A., Idler, E., Bjorner, J.B., Fayers, P.M. and Mouridsen, H.T. (2007) 'Psychological distress and fatigue predicted recurrence and survival in primary breast cancer patients'. *Breast Cancer Research and Treatment*, 105(2): 209–19

Guite, H., Clark, C. and Ackrill, G. (2006) 'The impact of the physical and urban environment on mental wellbeing'. *Public Health*, 120(12): 1117–26

Gutknecht, L., Jacob, C., Strobel, A., Kriegebaum, C., Müller, J., Zeng, Y., Markert, C., Wendland, A.E.J., Mössner, A.R.R., Gross, C., Brocke, B. and Lesch, K. (2007) 'Tryptophan hydroxylase-2 gene variation influences personality traits and disorders related to emotional dysregulation'. *The International Journal of Neuropsychopharmacology*, 10(3): 309–20

Gutman, L. and Feinstein, L. (2008) *Children's Well-Being in Primary School: Pupil and School Effects. Wider benefits of Learning Research Report No.*

25. London: Institute of Education, Centre for Research on the Wider Benefits of Learning

Guyton, A.C. and Hall, J.E. (2006) *Textbook of Medical Physiology* (11th Ed). Philadelphia, PA: Elsevier

Habell, M. (2010) 'The dementia care building crisis'. *Perspectives in Public Health*, 130(3):110

Hall, J.A., Carter, J.D. and Horgan, T.G. (2000) 'Gender differences in nonverbal communication of emotion' (pp. 97–117), in Fischer, A.H. (ed) *Gender and Emotion: social psychological perspectives*. Cambridge: Cambridge University Press

Halliday, J. (2010) *ADHD could be Linked to Diet: cohort study*. Available at **www.foodnavigator.com/Science-Nutrition/ADHD-could-be-linked-to-diet-Cohort-study** (accessed 15 August 2011)

Ham, C. (2009) *Health Policy in Britain*. London: Macmillan

Hansson, G.K. (2005) 'Inflammation, atherosclerosis and coronary artery disease'. *New England Journal of Medicine*, 352(16): 1685–95

Hart, A. (2008) 'Resilience and Well Being'. A presentation given to the East Sussex County Council Inclusive Learning team on 10 December 2008

Hassan, E., Austin C., Celia, C., Disley, E., Hunt, P., Marjanovic, S., Shehabi, A., Villalba-Van-Dijk, L. and Van Stolk, C. (2009) Health and Wellbeing at Work in the United Kingdom. London: The Work Foundation. Available at **www.nhshealthandwellbeing.org/pdfs/Interim%20Report%20Appendices/Literature%20Review.pdf** (accessed 15 August 2011)

Hastings, M.H., Reddy, A.B. and Maywood, E.S. (2003) 'A clockwork web: circadian timing in brain and periphery in health and disease'. *Nature Reviews Neuroscience*, 4: 641–61

Hatfield, B.D. (1991) 'Exercise and mental health: the mechanisms of exercise-induced psychological states' (pp. 17–50), in Diamant, L. (ed) *Psychology of Sports, Exercise and Fitness*. Washington, DC: Hemisphere

Hatfield, B.D. and Kaplan, P. (2004) 'Exercise psychology for the personal trainer' (pp. 142–58), in Earle, R.W. and Baechle, T.R. (eds) *NSCA's Essentials of Personal Training*. Champaign, IL: Human Kinetics

Haybron, D. (2008) *The Pursuit of Unhappiness*. Gloucestershire: Clarendon Press

Heart of Mersey (2005) *Food and Health Strategy for Greater Merseyside 2005*. Available at **www.heartofmersey.org.uk/cms_useruploads/files/greater_merseyside_food_and_health_strategy.pdf** (accessed 15 August 2011)

Helman, C.G. (1994) *Culture, Health and Illness*. Bristol: John Wright

Hernandez-Reif, M., Ironson, G., Field, T., Hurley, J., Katz, G., Diego, M., Weiss, S., Fletcher, M., Schanberg, S., Kuhn, C. and Burman, I. (2004) 'Breast cancer patients have improved immune and neuroendocrine functions following massage therapy'. *Journal of Psychosomatic Research*, 57(1): 45–52

Herzlinger, R. (1997) *Market Driven Healthcare: who wins, who loses in the transformation of America's largest service industry*. Massachusetts: Perseus Books

Higher Education Funding Council for England (HEFCE) (2010) The Higher Education Workforce Framework 2010 Main Report. Available at **www.hefce.ac.uk/pubs/hefce/2010/10_05a/10_05a.pdf** (accessed 15 August 2011)

Hirsch, A., Bartholomae, C. and Volmer, T. (2000) 'Dimensions of quality of life in people with non-insulin dependent diabetes'. *Quality of Life Research*, 9: 207–18

Hirschhorn, E., Haskins, R. and Nightingale, M. (2008) *Using the Media to Promote Adolescent Wellbeing.* Princeton-Brookings. Available at **http://ccf.tc.columbia.edu/pdf/Children%20and%20Electronic%20Media_18_01_PolicyBrief.pdf** (accessed 15 August 2011)

HM Government (2008) *Creating Strong, Safe and Prosperous Communities.* London: DCLG

HM Government (2010) *New Horizons, Confident Communities, Brighter Futures: a framework for developing well-being.* Available at **www.nmhdu.org.uk/silo/files/confident-communities-brighter-futures.pdf** (accessed 15 August 2011)

HMSO (2000) Local Government Act. London: HMSO

HM Treasury (2004) *Developments in the Economics of Wellbeing. Treasury economic working paper no: 4.* London: HM Treasury

Hofstader, R. (1992) *Social Darwinism and American Thought.* Philadelphia: University of Pennsylvania Press

Hogg, M. and Vaughan, G. (2005) *Social Psychology* (4th Ed). London: Prentice Hall

Holmes, E. (1911) *What Is and What Might Be.* London: Constable

House of Commons (2006) *Tackling Child Obesity – first steps* (HC 801 Session 2005–2006). London: The Stationery Office. (Accessed 19 May 2011)

House of Commons Communities and Local Government Committee (2009) *The Balance of Power: Central and Local Government Sixth Report of Session 2008–09 Report, together with formal minutes.* London: House of Commons, 12 May

House of Commons Health Committee (2004) *Obesity. Third report of session 2003–04 (HC23-1 27 May 2004).* London: The Stationery Office

Hsiung, P.C., Pan, A.W., Liu, S.K., Chen, S.C., Peng, S.Y. and Chung, L., (2010) 'Mastery and stigma in predicting the subjective quality of life of patients with schizophrenia in Taiwan'. *Journal of Nervous and Mental Disease*, 198(7): 494–500

Hui, L., Hua, F., Diandong, H. and Hong, Y. (2007) 'Effects of sleep and sleep deprivation on immunoglobulins and complement in humans'. *Brain Behaviour and Immunity*, 21: 308–10

Huppert, F.A. and Bayliss, N. (2004) 'Well-being: towards an integration of psychology, neurobiology and social science'. *Philosophical Transactions of the Royal Society, London B*, 359: 1447–51

Huppert, F.A., Marks, N., Clark, A.E., Siegrist, J., Stutzer, A., Vittersø, J. and Wahrendorf, M. (2008) *Measuring well-being across Europe: description of the ESS Well-being Module and preliminary findings. Working Paper No. 2008–40.* Paris: Paris School of Economics

Hursthouse, R. (1999) *On Virtue Ethics*. Maidenhead: Open University Press

Idea Store (2006) Available at **www.ideastore.co.uk** (accessed 15 August 2011)

Illich, I. (2001) *Limits to Medicine: medical nemesis – the expropriation of health*. London: Marion Boyes Publishers

International Diabetes Federation (IDF) (2005) *IDF Clinical Guidelines Task Force. Global guideline for Type 2 diabetes*. Brussels: International Diabetes Federation

International Diabetes Federation (IDF) (2005) *Worldwide Definition of the Metabolic Syndrome*. Available at **www.idf.org/webdata/docs/MetSyndrome_FINAL.pdf** (accessed 15 August 2011)

Irwin, M. (2002) 'Effects of sleep and sleep loss on immunity and cytokines'. *Brain Behaviour and Immunity*, 16(5): 503–12

Irwin, R.A., Davis, M. and Zautra, Z. (2008) 'Behavioural comorbidities in rheumatoid arthritis: a psychoneuroimmunological perspective'. *Psychiatric Times*, 25(9): 1–9

Jakobsson, U., Kristensson, J., Hallberg, I.G. and Midlov, P. (2010) 'Psychosocial perspectives on health care utilisation among frail elderly people: an explorative study'. *Archives of Gerontology and Geriatrics*, 4:16

Janki Foundation for Global Health Care (2004) 'Values in Healthcare: a spiritual approach: a personal and team development programme for healthcare practitioners'. Available at **www.jankifoundation.org/values_in_healthcare** (accessed 15 August 2011)

Jawień, J. (2008) 'New insights into immunological aspects of atherosclerosis'. *Polskie Archiwum Medycyny Wewnetrznej*,118(3): 127–31

Jiang, Y., Wilk, J.B., Borecki, I., Williamson, S., DeStefano, A.L., Xu, G., Liu, J., Ellison, R.C., Province, M. and Myers, R.H. (2004) 'Common Variants in the 5′ region of the leptin gene are associated with Body Mass index in men from the National Heart, Lung, and Blood Institute Family Heart Study'. *The American Journal of Human Genetics*, 75(2): 220–30

Johnson, D. and Tuttle, F. (1989) 'Problems in intercultural research', in Asante, M. and Gudykunst, W. (eds) *Handbook of International and Intercultural Communication*. California: Sage Publications

Joint Committee on Human Rights (2008) *A Bill of Rights for the UK?* 29th Report of Session 2007–08. HL Paper 165 – I/HC 150 – I. Available at **www.publications.parliament.uk/pa/jt200708/jtselect/jtrights/165/165i.pdf** (accessed 15 August 2011)

Jones-Devitt, S. and Smith, L. (2007) *Critical Thinking in Health and Social Care*. London: Sage Publications

Kabat-Zinn, J. (2003) 'Mindfulness-based interventions in context: past, present, and future'. *Clinical Psychology: Science and Practice*, 10: 144–56

Kagawa-Singer, M., Padilla, G.V. and Ashing-Giwa, K. (2010) 'Health-related quality of life and culture'. *Seminars in Oncology Nursing*, 261(1): 59–67

Kahneman, D., Diener, E. and Schwartz, N. (eds) (1999) *Well-being: the foundations of hedonic psychology*. New York: The Russell Age Foundation

Kawabata, A., Matsunami, M. and Sekiguchi, F. (2008) 'Gastrointestinal roles for proteinase-activated receptors in health and disease'. *British Journal of Pharmacology*, 153(1): 230–40

Kayani, N. (2009) 'Food, health and wellbeing', in Stewart, J. and Cornish, Y. (eds) *Professional Practice in Public Health*. Exeter: Reflect Press Ltd

Kelly, S.J., Ostrowski, N.L. and Wilson, M.A. (1999) 'Gender differences in brain and behaviour: hormonal and neural bases'. *Pharmacology Biochemistry and Behaviour*, 64(4): 655–64

Kiefer, R.A. (2008) 'An integrative review of the concept of wellbeing'. *Holistic Nursing Practice*, 22(5): 242–52

Kinder, A., Hughes, R. and Cooper, C.L. (2008) *Employee Wellbeing Support: a workplace resource*. West Sussex: Wiley and Sons

King's Fund (2003) *Health in the News*. London: King's Fund

Kirk, A.F., Higgins, L.A., Hughes, A.R., Fisher, M. B., Mutrie, N., Hillis, S. and MacIntyre, P.D. (2001) 'A randomized, controlled trial to study the effect of exercise consultation on the promotion of physical activity in people with Type 2 diabetes: a pilot study'. *Diabetic Medicine*, 18(11): 877–82

Kirk, A.F., Mutrie, N., Macintyre, P.D. and Fisher, M.B. (2004) 'Promoting and maintaining physical activity in people with type 2 diabetes'. *American Journal of Preventive Medicine*, 27(4): 289–96

Kleiman, A. (1988) *The Illness Narratives*. New York: Basic Books

Koenig, H.G. , McCullough, M.E. and Larson, D.B. (2001) *Handbook of Religion and Health*. Oxford: Oxford University Press

Konu, A. and Rimpelä, M. (2002) 'Well-being in schools: a conceptual model'. *Health Promotion International*, 17(1): 79–87

Koontz, H., O'Donnel, C. and Weirich, H. (1982) *Essentials of Management*. New Delhi: Tata, McGraw-Hill

Kop, W.J., Weissman, N.J., Zhu, J., Bonsall, R.W., Doyle, M., Stretch, M.R., Glaes, S.B., Krantz, D.S., Gottdiener, J.S. and Tracy, R.P. (2008) 'Effects of acute mental stress and exercise on inflammatory markers in patients with coronary artery disease and healthy controls'. *American Journal of Cardiology*, 101(6): 767–73

Kraut, R. (2007) *What is Good and Why*. Cambridge, MA: Harvard University Press

Kugler, J., Seelback, H. and Kruskemper, G.M. (1994) 'Effects of rehabilitation exercise programmes on anxiety and depression in coronary patients: a meta-analysis'. *British Journal of Clinical Psychology*, 33: 401–10

Kuppens, P., Realo, A. and Diener, E. (2008) 'The role of positive and negative emotions in life satisfaction judgement across nations'. *Journal of Personality and Social Psychology*, 95(1): 66–75

Kusel, J. (1996) 'Well-being in forest-dependent communities. Part I: a new approach' (pp. 361–73), in Sierra Nevada Ecosystem Project. *Sierra Nevada Ecosystem Project final report to Congress: status of the Sierra Nevada*. Davis, CA: Centers for Water and Wildland Resources, University of California

Kvaskoff, M. and Weinstein, P. (2010) 'Are some melanomas caused by artificial light?' *Medical Hypotheses*, 75(3): 305–311

Kwan, C.M.L., Love, G.D., Ryff, C.D. and Essex, M.J. (2003) 'The role of self-enhancing evaluation in a successful life transition'. *Psychological Ageing*, 19: 3–12

Lancet (1991) Consanguinity and Health. *The Lancet*, 338: 85–6

Landers, D.M. and Arent, S.A. (2001) 'Physical activity and mental health' (pp. 740–65) in Singer, R.N., Hausenblas, H.A. and Janelle, C.M. (eds) *Handbook of Sport Psychology* (2nd Ed). New York: Wiley

Landers, D.M. and Petruzzello, S.J. (1994) 'Physical activity, fitness and anxiety' (pp. 868–82), in Bouchard, C., Shepard, R.J and Stevens, T. (eds) *Physical Activity, Fitness, and Health* (4th Ed). Champaign, IL: Human Kinetics

Larson, E.T. and Summers, C.H. (2001) 'Serotonin reverses dominant social status'. *Behavioural Brain Research*, 121(1–2): 95–102

Lawrence, F. (2010) 'Good for the nation's health – or for big business?' *The Guardian*, 13 November: 4

Layard, R. (2005) *Happiness: lessons from a new science*. London: Allen Lane

Lazenbatt, A., Orr, J. and O'Neill, E. (2001) 'Inequalities in health: evaluation and effectiveness in practice'. *International Journal of Nursing Practice*, 7 (6): 383–91

Leacock, E.B. (1971) *The Culture of Poverty: a critique*. New York: Simon & Schuster

Leeds University (2010a) Latest News: Wellbeing Team wins £350,000 HEFCE Bid. Available at **www.wellbeing.leeds.ac.uk** (accessed 15 August 2011)

Leeds University (2010b) *Wellbeing Strategy*. Available at **www.wellbeing. leeds.ac.uk/our-aim/** (accessed 15 August 2011)

Leidy, N.K., Revicki, D.A. and Geneste, B. (1999) 'Recommendations for evaluating the validity of quality of life claims for labeling and promotion'. *Value Health*, 2(2): 113–27

Leonard, B. (2000) 'Stress, depression and the activation of the immune system'. *World Journal of Biological Psychiatry*, 1(1): 17–25

Lesperance, F. *et al.* (2010) 'The efficacy of omega-3 supplementation for major depression: a randomised controlled trial'. *Journal of Clinical Psychiatry*, abstract only. Available at **www.ncbi.nlm.nih.gov/pubmed/20584525** (accessed 15 August 2011)

Levy, B., Slade, M., Kunkel, S. and Kasl, S. (2002) 'Longevity increased by positive self perceptions of aging'. *Journal of Personality and Social Psychology*, 83(2): 261–70

Lewis, O. (1961) *The Children of Sanchez: autobiography of a Mexican family*. New York: Random House

Libby, P., Okamoto, Y., Rocha, V.Z. and Folco, E. (2010) 'Inflammation in atherosclerosis: transition from theory to practice'. *Circulation Journal*, 74(2): 213–20

Liebregts, T., Adam, B., Bredack, C., Röth, A., Heinzel, S., Lester, S., Downie-Doyle, S., Smith, E., Drew, P., Talley, N.J. and Holtmann, G. (2007) 'Immune activation in patients with irritable bowel syndrome'. *Gastroenterology*, 132(3): 913–20

Lindblom, C. (1979) 'Still muddling: not yet through'. *Public Administration Review*, 39: 517–26

Lindfors, P., Berntsson, L. and Lundberg, U. (2006) 'Factor structure of Ryff's psychological well-being scales in Swedish female and male white-collar workers'. *Personality and Individual Differences*, 40: 1213–22

Lister, S., Perry, J. and Thornley, M. (2007) *Community Engagement in Housing-Led Regeneration: a good practice guide.* Coventry: CIH and TPAS

Lloyd-Williams, F. and Mair, F. (2005) 'The role of exercise in recovery from heart failure' (pp. 70–96), in Faulkner, G. and Taylor, A.H. (eds) *Exercise, Health and Mental Health: emerging relationships.* London: Routledge

Long, B.C. and Van Stavel, R. (1995) 'Effects of exercise training on anxiety: a meta-analysis'. *Journal of Applied Sports Psychology*, 7: 167–89

Love, K., Pritchard, C., Maguire, K., McCarthy, A. and Paddock, P. (2005) 'Qualitative and quantitative approaches to health impact assessment: an analysis of the political and philosophical milieu of the multi-method approach'. *Critical Public Health*, 15(3): 275–89

Lowe, M.R. and Butryn, M.L. (2007) 'Hedonic hunger: a new dimension of appetite?' *Physiology & Behaviour*, 91(4): 432–9

Lukes, S. (1978) *Power.* London: Macmillan

Lundberg, A.M. and Hansson, G.K. (2010) 'Innate immune signals in atherosclerosis'. *Clinical Immunology*, 134(1): 5–24

Lynd, R. and Morrell, H. (1929) *Middletown.* New York: Harcourt, Brace and Jovanovich

Lynd, R. and Morrell, H. (1937) *Middletown in Transition.* New York: Harcourt, Brace and Jovanovich

Lyubomirsky, S., King, L. and Diener, E. (2005) 'The benefits of frequent positive affect: does happiness lead to success?' *Psychological Bulletin*, 131(6): 803–55

Macintyre, A. (2007) *After Virtue: a study in moral theory* (3rd Ed). London: Gerald Duckworth & Co.

MacIntyre, P.D. (2001) 'A randomized, controlled trial to study the effect of exercise consultation on the promotion of physical activity in people with Type 2 diabetes: a pilot study'. *Diabetes Medicine*, 18(11): 877–82

MacKerron, G. and Mourato, S. (2009) 'Life satisfaction and air quality in London'. *Ecological Economics*, 68(5): 1441–53

Maddigan, S.L., Feeny, D.H., Majumdar, S.R., Farris, K.B. and Johnson, J.A. (2006) 'Understanding the determinants of health in Type 2 Diabetes'. *American Journal of Public Health*, 96(9):1649–55

Manglalasche, F., Kivipelto, M., Mecocci, P., Rizzuto, D., Palmer, K., Winblad, B. and Fratiglioni, L. (2010) 'High plasma levels of vitamin E forms and reduced Alzheimer's disease risk in advanced age'. *Journal of Alzheimer's Disease*, abstract only. Available at **www.ncbi.nlm.nih.gov/pubmed/20413888** (accessed 15 August 2011)

Marcus, B.H. and Simkin, L.R. (1994) 'The transtheoretical model: applications to exercise behavior'. *Medicine and Science in Sports and Exercise*, 26(11): 1400–4

Marinoff, L. (1999) *Plato not Prozac: applying eternal wisdom to everyday problems.* London: HarperCollins

Marks, N. (2005) 'Wellbeing and Social Policy'. Given at Social Policy Association Conference, University of Bath. 29 June. Available at **www.bath.ac.uk/soc-pol/.../spa.../wellbeing-and-public-policy-n-marks.ppt** (accessed 15 August 2011)

Marmot, M., Allen, J., Goldblatt, P., Boyce, T., McNeish, D., Grady, M., *et al.* (2010) *Fair Society, Healthy Lives. The Marmot Review. Strategic Review of Health Inequalities in England post-2010.* London: Department of Health

Martinez-Lavin, M., Infante, C. and Lerma, C. (2008) 'Hypotheses: the chaos and complexity theory may help our understanding of fibromyalgia and other similar maladies'. *Seminars in Arthritis and Rheumatism,* 37(4): 260–4

Mattson, M.P., Maudsley, S. and Bronwen, M. (2004) 'BDNF and 5-HT: a dynamic duo in age-related neuronal plasticity and neurodegenerative disorders'. *Trends in Neurosciences,* 27(10): 589–94

Maxwell, C. and Warwick, I. (2007) 'Student mental health and wellbeing in further education'. Learning for Life. **www.teachingexpertise.com/articles/student-mental-health-and-wellbeing-1593** (accessed 15 August 2011)

McCallum, I. (2005) *Ecological Intelligence: rediscovering ourselves in nature.* Cape Town, South Africa: Africa Geographic Books

McCawley, P. (1997) *The Logic Model for Program Planning and Evaluation.* Idaho: University of Idaho

McCloud, K. (2008) *Kevin McCloud and the Big Town Plan.* Available at **www.channel4.com/4homes/on-tv/kevin-s-big-town-plan** (accessed 15 August 2011)

McCormick, B. and Stone, I. (2007) 'Economic costs of obesity and the case for government intervention'. *Obesity Reviews* 8(1):161–4

McDonald, D.G. and Hodgdon, J.A. (1991) *The Psychological Effects of Aerobic Fitness Training: Research and Theory.* New York: Springer-Verlag

McGhee, P. (2010) *Humour: the lighter path to resilience and health.* Bloomingtom, IN: Author House

Medway Council (2010) Wellbeing Service in Medway. Available at **www.medway.gov.uk/educationandlearning/informationforschools/leadershipandmanagement/healthyschools/staffwellbeing.aspx** (accessed 15 August 2011)

Meeus, M., Mistiaen, W., Lambrecht, L. and Nijs, J. (2009) 'Immunological similarities between cancer and chronic fatigue syndrome: the common link to fatigue?' *Anticancer Research,* 29(11): 4717–26

Meijer, E, Goris, A., Van Dongen, J., Bast, A. and Westerterp, K. (2002) 'Exercise-induced oxidative stress in older adults as a function of habitual activity level'. *Journal of the American Geriatrics Society,* 50(2): 349–53

Ménard, J., Payette, H., Dubuc, N., Baillargeon, J.P., Maheux, P. and Ardilouze, J.L. (2007) 'Quality of life in type 2 diabetes patients under intensive multitherapy'. *Diabetes and Metabolism,* 33(1): 54–60

Mental Health Foundation (2007) *Making Space for Spirituality: how to support service users.* London: Mental Health Foundation

Milburn, K. (1996) 'The importance of lay theorizing for health promotion theory and practice'. *Health Promotion International,* 11: 1–46

Mind (2007) *Ecotherapy: The Green Agenda for Mental Health*. Available at **www.mind.org.uk/assets/0000/2138/ecotherapy_report.pdf** (accessed 15 August 2011)

More, T. (1516) *Utopia*. Available at **http://oregonstate.edu/instruct/phl302/texts/more/utopia-I.html** (accessed 15 August 2011)

Moreno-Leguizamon, C. (2005) 'Dichotomies in Western biomedicine and Ayurveda: health-illness and body-mind'. *Economic and Political Weekly*, 40(30): 3302–10

Morgan, W.P. (1985) 'Affective beneficence of vigorous physical activity'. *Medicine and Science in Sports and Exercise*, 17: 94–100

Morikawa, Y., Kitaoka-Higashiguchi, K., Tanimoto, C., Hayashi, M., Oketani, R., Miura. K., Nishijo, M. and Nakagawa, H. (2005) 'A cross-sectional study on the relationship of job stress with natural killer cell activity and natural killer cell subsets among healthy nurses'. *Journal of Occupational Health*, 47: 378–83

Morin, C.M., Rodrigue, S. and Ivers, H. (2003) 'Role of stress, arousal, and coping skills in primary insomnia'. *Psychosomatic Medicine*, 65(2): 259–67

Morris, I. (2009) *Teaching Happiness and Wellbeing in Schools*. London: Continuum

Morrison, V. and Bennett, P. (2006) *An Introduction to Health Psychology*. Harlow: Pearson/Prentice Hall

Murphy, D.L. and Lesch, K.P. (2008) 'Targeting the murine serotonin transporter: insights into human neurobiology'. *Nature Reviews Neuroscience*, 9(2): 85–96

Nafstad, H.E., Blakar, R.M., Carlquist, E., Phelps, J.M. and Rand-Hendriksen, K. (2007) 'Ideology and power: the influence of current neo-liberalism in society'. *Journal of Community and Applied Social Psychology*, 17: 313–27

Nakamura, M., Ueno, S., Sano, A. and Tanabe, H. (2000) 'The human serotonin transporter gene linked polymorphism (5-HTTLPR) shows ten novel allelic variants'. *Molecular Psychiatry*, 5(1): 32

National Institute for Health and Clinical Excellence (NICE) (2004) *Improving Supportive and Palliative Care for Adults: the manual*. London: NICE

National Institute for Health and Clinical Excellence (NICE) (2008) *Mental Wellbeing and Older People: guidance for occupational therapy and physical activity interventions to promote the mental wellbeing of older people in primary care and residential care*. Available at **www.nice.org.uk/nicemedia/pdf/PH16guidance.pdf** (accessed 15 August 2011)

Natural England (2008) *Natural England's Position on Health and Wellbeing*. Available at **http://www.naturalengland.org.uk/Images/draftpolicyonhealthandwellbeing0907_tcm6-3699.pdf** (accessed 15 August 2011)

Natural England (2009) *Natural Health Service Concordat*. Available at **www.naturalengland.org.uk/Images/NHSconcordat_tcm6-12517.pdf** (accessed 15 August 2011)

Natural England (2010) *Monitor of Engagement with the Natural Environment: The National Survey on People and the Natural Environment. Annual Report from the 2009–10 Survey. NECR049.* Available at **http://naturalengland. etraderstores.com/NaturalEnglandShop/NECR049** (accessed 15 August 2011)

Nettleton, S. (1995) *The Sociology of Health and Illness.* Cambridge: Polity Press

New Economics Foundation (NEF) (2004)*The Potential and Power of Wellbeing Indicators: measuring young people's wellbeing in Nottingham.* Available at **www.neweconomics.org/publications/power-and-potential-well-being-indicators** (accessed 15 August 2011)

New Economics Foundation (NEF) (2004) *A Well-Being Manifesto for a Flourishing Society.* London: NEF

New Economics Foundation (NEF) (2009) *National Accounts of Well-being: bringing real wealth onto the balance sheet.* London: NEF

Newton, J. (2007) *Wellbeing and the Natural Environment: a brief overview of the Evidence.* Available at **www3.surrey.ac.uk/resolve/seminars/Julie%20 Newton%20Paper.pdf** (accessed 15 August 2011)

NHS (2009a) *Health and Wellbeing Interim Report.* Available at **www. nhshealthandwellbeing.org/pdfs/NHS%20HWB%20Review%20 Interim%20Report%20190809.pdf** (accessed 15 August 2011)

NHS (2009b) *Health and Wellbeing Final Report.* Available at **www. nhshealthandwellbeing.org/pdfs/NHS%20Staff%20H&WB%20 Review%20Final%20Report%20VFinal%2020-11-09.pdf** (accessed 15 August 2011)

NHS (2009c) *NHS Health and Wellbeing: Staff Health and Wellbeing Case Studies.* Available at **www.nhshealthandwellbeing.org/pdfs/Staff%20 H&WB%20Case%20Studies%20VFinal%2023-11-09.pdf** (accessed 15 August 2011)

NHS (2010) *The NHS Constitution: The NHS Belongs to Us All.* Available at **www.dh.gov.uk/prod_consum_dh/groups/dh_digitalassets/@dh/@ en/@ps/documents/digitalasset/dh_113645.pdf** (accessed 26 August 2010)

NHS Education for Scotland (2009) *Spiritual Care Matters.* Edinburgh: NHS Education for Scotland

NHS Information Centre (2006) *Rise in Childhood Obesity Rates: new statistics from health survey for England, April 2005–March 2006.* Available at **www.ic.nhs.uk/news-and-events/press-office/press-releases/archived-press-releases/april-2005--march-2006/rise-in-childhood-obesity-rates--new-statistics-from-health-survey-for-england** (accessed 15 August 2011)

Nieman, D.C., Custer, W.F., Butterworth, D.E., Utter, A. and Henson, D.A. (2000) 'Psychological response to exercise training and/or energy restriction in obese women'. *Journal of Psychosomatic Research,* 48(1): 22–9

North, T.C., McCullagh, P. and Tran, V.Z. (1990) 'Effects of exercise on depression'. *Exercise and Sport Science Reviews,* 18: 379–415

Northern Housing Consortium (2010) *A Guide to Age Friendly Communities in the North: people and places 2020.* Sunderland: Northern Housing Consortium

Nowakowski, L.A.E. (2007) *Increasing the Reliability of Wellness Metrics in Unique Groups.* Thailand: Ubon Ratchathani University

Nozick, R. (1974) *Anarchy, State and Utopia*. USA: Basic Books

Nurse, J., Basher, D., Bone, A. and Bird, W. (2010) 'An ecological approach to promoting population mental health and well-being: a response to the challenge of climate change'. *Perspectives in Public Health*, 130(1): 27–33

Nussbaum, M.C. (1994) *The Therapy of Desire: theory and practice in Hellenistic ethics*. Princeton, NJ: Princeton University Press

Nybo, L. and Secher, N.H. (2004) 'Cerebral perturbations provoked by prolonged exercise'. *Progress in Neurobiology*, 72(4): 223–61

O'Brien, L. (2006) 'Strengthening heart and mind: using woodlands to improve mental and physical well-being'. *Unasylva*, 57: 224. Available at **www.fao.org/docrep/009/a0789e/a0789e00.htm** (accessed 15 August 2011)

O'Brien, L. and Morris, J. (2009) *Active England. The Woodland Projects*. Available at **www.forestresearch.gov.uk/pdf/active_england_final_report.pdf/$FILE/active_england_final_report.pdf** (accessed 15 August 2011)

O'Brien, M. (1995) 'Health and lifestyle: a critical mess?' (Chapter 15, pp. 191–205), in Bunton, R., Nettleton, S. and Burrows, R. (eds) *The Sociology of Health Promotion: critical analyses of consumption, lifestyle and risk*. London: Routledge

O'Donovan, A., Lin, J., Dhabhar, F.S., Wolkowitz, O., Tillie, J.M. and Blackburn, E. (2009) 'Pessimism correlates with leukocyte telomere shortness and elevated interleukin–6 in post-menopausal women'. *Brain Behaviour & Immunity*, 23: 446–9

Offer, A., Pechey, R. and Ulijaszek, S. (2010) 'Obesity under affluence varies by welfare regimes: the effect of fast food, insecurity and inequality'. *Discussion Papers in Economic and Social History*, Economics and Human Biology (In press)

Office for National Statistics (ONS) (2003) *Religious Populations*. Available at **www.statistics.gov.uk/cci/nugget.asp?id=954** (accessed 15 August 2011)

Office of Public Sector Information (2010) Local Government Act 2000. Available at **www.opsi.gov.uk/Acts/acts2000/ukpga_20000022_en_1** (accessed 15 August 2011)

Office of the Deputy Prime Minister (ODPM) (2003) *Sustainable Communities: building for the future*. London: HMSO

Office of the Deputy Prime Minister (2004) *Decent Homes: definition and guidance for implementation*. London: HMSO

Office of the Deputy Prime Minister (ODPM) (2005) *Sustainable Communities: people, places and prosperity*. Available at **www.communities.gov.uk/documents/corporate/pdf/people-places-prosperity.pdf** (accessed 15 August 2011)

Office of the Deputy Prime Minister (ODPM) (2005a) *Living Places: cleaner, safer, greener*. Available at **www.communities.gov.uk/publications/communities/livingplacescleaner** (accessed 15 August 2011)

Oishi, S., Schimmack, U., Diener, E., Kim-Prieto, C., Scollon, C.N. and Choi, D.W. (2007) 'The value-congruence model of memory for emotional experiences: an explanation for cultural differences in emotional self-reports. *Journal of Personality and Social Psychology*, 93(5): 899–905

O'Leary, A. (1990) 'Stress, emotion, and human immune function'. *Psychological Bulletin*, 108(3): 363–82

O'Leary, J.V. (2008) 'Putting it together while falling apart: a personal view on depression'. *Contemporary Psychoanalysis*, 44: 531–55

Olson, R.E. (1998) 'Discovery of the lipoproteins, their role in fat transport and their significance as risk factors'. *The Journal of Nutrition*, 128(2): 439S–443S

Olssen, M. and Peters, M.A. (2005) 'Neoliberalism, higher education and the knowledge economy: from the free market to knowledge capitalism'. *Journal of Educational Policy*, 20(3): 313–45

Organisation for Economics Cooperation and Development (OECD) (2000) *Results-based Management in the Development Cooperation Agencies: a review of experience*. Paris: Development Cooperation Directorate

Orme, J., DeViggiani, N., Naidoo, J. and Knight, T. (2007) 'Missed opportunities? Locating health promotion within multidisciplinary public health'. *Public Health*, 121: 414–19

Pacione, M. (2003) 'Urban environmental quality and human wellbeing – a social geographic perspective'. *Landscape and Urban Planning*, 65: 19–30

Page, C. (1998) 'The spirit in practice'. *Complementary Therapies in Nursing and Midwifery*, (4): 100–3

Pan, X.R., Li, G.W., Hu, Y.H., Wang, J.X., Yang, W.Y., An, Z.X., Hu, Z.X., Lin, J., Xiao, J.Z., Cao, H.B., Liu, P.A., Jiang, X.G., Wang, J.P., Zheng, H., Zhang, H., Bennet, P.H. and Howard, B.V. (1997) 'Effects of diet and exercise in preventing NIDDM in people with impaired glucose tolerance: the Da Qing IGT and Diabetes Study'. *Diabetes Care*, 20: 537–44

Parfit, D. (1984) *Reasons and Persons*. Oxford: Oxford University Press

Pedersen, B.K. and Saltin, B. (2006) 'Evidence for prescribing exercise as therapy in chronic disease'. *Journal of Sports Science and Medicine*, 1: 3–63

Peirano, P., Algarín, C. and Uauy, R. (2003) 'Sleep-wake states and their regulatory mechanisms throughout early human development'. *Journal of Paediatrics*, 143(4): 70–9

Pert, C.B. (1999) *Molecules of Emotion*. London: Simon and Schuster

Pert, C.B., Dreher, H.E. and Ruff, M.R. (1998) 'The psychosomatic network: foundations of mind-body medicine'. *Alternative Therapies*, 4(4): 30–41

Pert, C.B., Ruff, M.R., Weber, R.J. and Herkenham, M. (1985) 'Neuropeptides and their receptors: a psychosomatic network'. *Journal of Immunology*, 135 (Suppl 2): 820–6

Petruzzello, S.J., Landers, D.M., Hatfield, K.A., Kubitz, K.A. and Salazar, W. (1991) 'A meta-analysis on the anxiety-reduction effects of acute and chronic exercise'. *Sports Medicine*, 11:143–82

Physical Activity Guidelines Advisory Committee (2008) *Physical Activity Guidelines Advisory Committee Report, 2008*. Washington, DC: US Department of Health and Human Services

Pickett, K.E., Kelly, S., Leach, R., Brunner, E. and Wilkinson, R.G. (2005) 'Wider income gaps, wider waistbands? An ecological study of income inequality and obesity'. *Journal of Epidemiology and Community Health*, 59: 670–4

Pierson, C. (1996) *The Modern State*. London: Routledge

Pinquart, M. and Sorensen, S. (2001) 'How effective are psychotherapeutic and other psychosocial interventions with older adults?' *Journal of Mental Health and Aging*, 7(2): 207–43

Plato (1992) *Republic*, Hackett cited in Haybron, D. (2008) *The Pursuit of Unhappiness*. Oxford: Clarendon Press

Plum Village (2010) Art of Mindful Living: breathing. Available at **www.plumvillage.org/practice.html?start=4** (accessed 15 August 2011)

Politi, P.L., Piccinelli, M. and Wilkinson, G. (1994) 'Reliability, validity and factor structure of the 12-item General Health Questionnaire among young males in Italy'. *Acta Psychiatrica Scandinavica*, 90(6): 432–7

Praet, S.F., van Rooij, E.S., Wijtvliet, A., Boonman-de Winter, L.J., Enneking, T., Kuipers, H., Stehouwer, C.D. and van Loon, L.J. (2008) 'Brisk walking compared with an individualised medical fitness programme for patients with type 2 diabetes: a randomised controlled trial'. *Diabetologia*, 51(5): 736–46

PriceWaterhouseCooper (2008) Building the Case for Wellness. Available at **www.workingforhealth.gov.uk/documents/dwp-wellness-report-public.pdf** (accessed 15 August 2011)

Programme for International Student Assessment (PISA) (2010) *PISA 2009 Results: What students know and can do: student performance in reading, mathematics and science. Vol 1*. Paris: OECD

Rachels, J. (1999) *The Elements of Moral Philosophy*. New York: McGraw-Hill International

Raglin, J.S., Wilson, G.S. and Galper, D. (2007) 'Exercise and its effects on mental health' (pp. 157–83) in Bouchard, C., Blair, S. and Haskell, W. (eds) *Physical Activity and Health*. Champaign, IL: Human Kinetics

Ramachandran, A., Snehalatha, C., Mary, S., Mukesh, B., Bhaskar, A.D. and Vijay, V. (2006) 'Indian Diabetes Prevention Programme (IDPP).The Indian Diabetes Prevention Programme shows that lifestyle modification and metformin prevent type 2 diabetes in Asian Indian subjects with impaired glucose tolerance (IDPP-1)'. *Diabetologia*, 49(2): 289–97

Ranjit, N., Young, E.A., Raghunathan, T.E. and Kaplan, G.A. (2005) 'Modelling cortisol rhythms in a population-based study'. *Psychoneuroimmunology*, 30: 615–24

Rapps, N., Oudenhove, L., Enck, P. and Aziz, Q. (2008) 'Brain imaging of visceral functions in healthy volunteers and IBS patients'. *Journal of Psychosomatic Research*, 64: 599–604

Rath, T. and Harter, J. (2010) *Wellbeing: the five essential elements*. New York: Gallup Press

Raz, J. (2004) 'The role of wellbeing'. *Philosophical Perspectives*, 18: 269–94

Rehdanz, K. and Maddison, D. (2006) *Local Environmental Quality and Life-Satisfaction in Germany. Working paper FNU-119*. Available at **http://fnu.zmaw.de/fileadmin/fnu-files/publication/working-papers/FNU-119.pdf** (accessed 15 August 2011)

Reigelman, R. (2010) *Public Health 101: healthy people, healthy populations*. UK: Jones & Bartlett

Rejeski, W.J., Lang, W., Neiberg, R.H., Van Dorsten, B., Foster, G.D., Maciejewski, M.L., Rubin, R. and Williamson, D.F. Look AHEAD Research Group (2006) 'Correlates of health-related quality of life in overweight and obese adults with type 2 diabetes'. *Obesity*, 14(5): 870–83

Rettig, K.D. and Leichtentritt, R.D. (1999) 'A general theory for perceptual indicators of family life quality'. *Social Indicators Research*, 47: 307–42. In Wollny *et al.* (2010)

Rhoden, M. (forthcoming) *Housing and Social Policy: an introduction*. London: Routledge

Ridge, D., Williams, I., Anderson, J. and Elford, J. (2008) 'Like a prayer: the role of spirituality and religion for people living with HIV in the UK'. *Sociology of Health and Illness*, 30(3): 413–28

Robinson, J. (2010) 'The business case for wellbeing: having high levels of wellbeing is good for people – and their employers'. *Podcast-Gallup Management Journal*, 9 June 2010

Rosenwasser, A.M. (2009) 'Functional neuroanatomy of sleep and circadian rhythm'. *Brain Research Review*: 281–306

Royal College of Psychiatrists (RCP) (2003) *The Mental Health of Students In Higher Education – Council Report 112*. Available at **www.rcpsych.ac.uk/publications/collegereports/cr/cr112.aspx** (accessed 15 August 2011)

Royal Commission on Environmental Pollution (2007) *The Urban Environment. Twenty-Sixth Report*. Available at **www.rcep.org.uk/reports/26-urban/documents/urban-environment.pdf** (accessed 15 August 2011)

Ruini, C. and Fava, G.A. (2009) 'Well-being therapy for generalized anxiety disorder'. *Journal of Clinical Psychology*, 65(5): 510–19

Rundall, T.G. and Wheeler, J.R.C. (1979) 'The effect of income on the use of preventive care: an evaluation of alternative explanations'. *Journal of Health and Social Behavior*, 20: 397–406

Ryan, R. and Deci, E.L. (2001) 'On happiness and human potentials: a review of research on hedonic and eudaimonic well-being'. *Annual Review of Psychology*, 52: 141–66

Ryckman, P. (2004) *Theories of Personality*. Belmont, CA: Thomson/Wadsworth

Ryff, C. (1989a) 'Beyond Ponce de Leon and life satisfaction: new directions in quest of successful aging'. *International Journal of Behavioural Development*, 12: 35–55

Ryff, C. (1989b) 'Happiness is everything or is it? Explorations on the meaning of psychological well-being'. *Journal of Personality and Social Psychology*, 57: 1069–81

Ryff, C.D. and Singer, B.H. (2008) 'Know thyself and become what you are: a eudaimonic approach to psychological well-being'. *Journal of Happiness Studies*, 9(1): 13–39

Saracci, R. (1997) 'The World Health Organization needs to reconsider its definition of health'. *British Medical Journal*, 314: 1409

Schickler, P. (2005) 'Achieving health or achieving wellbeing'. *Learning in Health and Social Care*, 4(4): 217–27

Schimmack. U., Oishi. S. and Diener, E. (2005) Individualism: a valid and important dimension of cultural differences between nations'. *Personality and Social Psychology Review,* 9(1): 17–31

Schneider, J., Murray, J., Banerjee, S. and Mann, A. (1999) 'Eurocare: a cross-sectional study of co-resident spouse carers for people with Alzheimer's disease: I-Factors associated with carer's burden'. *International Journal of Geriatric Psychiatry,* 14: 651–61

Scottish Government (2003) *Enhancing Sexual Wellbeing in Scotland: a sexual health relationship strategy.* Crown Copyright. Available at **www.scotland. gov.uk/Publications/2003/11/18503/28872** (accessed 15 August 2011)

Seedhouse, D. (1995) 'Wellbeing: health promotion's red herring'. *Health Promotion International,* 10(1): 61–7

Segal, Z.V., Williams, J.M.G. and Teasdale, J.D. (2002) *Mindfulness-based Cognitive Therapy for Depression: a new approach to preventing relapse.* New York: Guilford Press

Seifert, T.A. (2005) *The Ryff Scales of Psychological Well-Being.* Center of Inquiry, IN: Wabash College

Selznick, P. (1992) *The Moral Commonwealth: social theory and the promise of community.* California: University of California Press

Shah, H. and Marks, N. (2004) 'A wellbeing manifesto for a flourishing society'. *The Power of Wellbeing,* 3. London: New Economics Foundation

Shakhar, K., Valdimarsdottir, H.B., Guevarra, J.S. and Bovbjerg, D.H. (2007) 'Sleep, fatigue, and NK cell activity in healthy volunteers: significant relationships revealed by within subject analyses'. *Brain Behaviour and Immunity,* 21: 180–4

Shapiro, D.H., Schwartz, C.E. and Astin, J.A. (1996) 'Controlling ourselves, controlling our world'. *American Psychologist,* 51(12): 1213–23

Sherwood, D.E. and Selder, D.J. (1979) 'Cardiorespiratory health, reaction time and aging'. *Medicine and Science in Sports,* 11:186–9

Shishehbor, M.H. and Bhatt, D.L. (2004) 'Inflammation and atherosclerosis'. *Current Atherosclerosis Reports,* 6(2): 131–9

Sibille, E. and Lewis, D.A. (2007) 'SERT-ainly involved in depression, but when?' *American Journal of Psychiatry,* 163: 8–11

Sigal, R.J., Wasserman, D.H., Kenny, G.P. and Castaneda, C. (2004) 'Physical Activity/Exercise and type 2 diabetes'. *Diabetes Care,* 10: 2518–39

Simon, H. (1957) *Administrative Behaviour.* London: Macmillan

Skilton, L. (2009) *Working Paper: Measuring Societal Wellbeing in the UK.* London: ONS

Slote, M. (2001) 'Virtue ethics', in Lafollette, H. (2001) *The Blackwell Guide to Ethical Theory.* Oxford: Blackwell Publishing

Smedley, B.D., Stith, A.Y. and Nelson, A.R. (2003) *Unequal Treatment: confronting racial and ethnic disparities in health care,* Washington, DC: National Academies Press

Snyder, C.R. and Lopez, S.J. (eds) *Handbook of Positive Psychology,* Chapter 3, pp. 63–73. New York: Oxford University Press

Social Exclusion Unit (SEU) (2001) *A New Commitment to Neighbourhood Renewal: National Strategy Action Plan.* Available at **www.neighbourhood. statistics.gov.uk/HTMLDocs/images/NationalStrategyReport_tcm97-51090.pdf** (accessed 15 August 2011)

Society for the Study of Ingestive Behaviour (2010) *A high fat diet alters crucial aspects of brain dopamine signaling* (press release 13 July 2010). Available at **www.ssib.org/web/index.php?page=press&release=2010-8** (accessed 15 August 2011)

Somers J.M., Goldner, E.M., Waraich, P. and Hsu, L. (2006) 'Prevalence and incidence studies of anxiety disorders: a systematic review of the literature'. *Canadian Journal of Psychiatry*, 51: 100–3

Speakman, J.R., Rance, K.A. and Johnstone, A.M. (2008) 'Polymorphisms of the FTO gene are associated with variation in energy intake, but not energy expenditure'. *Obesity*, 16(8):1961–5

Spear, S. (2008) *Fast food fears.* Available at **www.cieh.org/ehp/fast_food_fears.html** (accessed 15 August 2011)

Spear, S. (2010) *Fast food make-over.* Available at **www.cieh.org/ehn/ehn3.aspx?id=32140&terms=fast+food+make+over** (accessed 15 August 2011)

Spigner, C. (2006–7) 'Race, health, and the African diaspora'. *International Quarterly of Community Health Education*, 27(2): 161-76

Spoormaker, V.I. and Bout, J.V.D. (2005) 'Depression and anxiety complaints: relations with sleep disturbances'. *Department of Clinical Psychology*, 20: 243–54

Stainton Rogers, W. (1991) *Exploring Health and Illness: an exploration of diversity.* London: Harvester Wheatsheaf

Stansfeld, S. and Matheson, M. (2003) 'Noise pollution: non-auditory effects on health'. *British Medical Bulletin*, 68(1): 243–57

Starling, G. (1982) *Managing the Public Sector.* Illinois: The Dorsey Press

Stecker, T. (2004) 'Well-being in an academic environment'. *Medical Education*, 38(5): 465–78

Steptoe, A. (2006) *Depression and Physical Illness.* Cambridge: Cambridge University Press

Steptoe, A., O'Donnell, K., Badrick, E., Kumari, M. and Marmot, M. (2008) 'Neuroendocrine and inflammatory factors associated with positive affect in healthy men and women. The Whitehall II Study'. *American Journal of Epidemiology*, 167(1): 96–102

Steuer, N. and Marks, N. (2008) *University Challenge: towards a well-being approach to quality in higher education.* London: NEF

Stewart, J., Bushell, F. and Habgood, V. (2005) *Environmental Health as Public Health.* London: Chadwick House Group Ltd

Stiglitz, J.E. (2002) 'Employment, social justice and societal well-being'. *International Labour Review*, 141(1–2): 9–29

Stockdale, L. (2010) 'Forget me not'. *Inside Housing*, 12 February, pp. 38–9

Stone, A., Schwartz, J., Broderick, J. and Deaton, A. (2010) 'Stress, anger, and worry fade after 50'. *Proceedings of the National Academy of Sciences*, May, pp. 17–21

Stone, D. (2006) 'Sustainable development: convergence of public health and natural environment agendas, nationally and locally'. *Public Health*, 120(12): 1110–13

Stratton, A. (2010) *Happiness Index to Gauge Britain's National Mood.* London: *The Guardian*, 15 November

Stubbe, J.H., de Moor, M.H.M., Boomsma, D.I. and de Geus, E.J.C. (2007) 'The association between exercise participation and well-being: a co-twin study'. *Preventive Medicine*, 44(2): 148–52

Suarez-Herrera, J.C., Springett, J. and Kagan, C. (2009) 'Critical connections between participatory evaluation, organizational learning and intentional change in pluralistic organizations'. *Evaluation*, 15(3): 321–42

Sustainable Development Commission (2007) *Proposal for a Wellbeing Indicators Framework*. Available at **www.sd-commission.org.uk/sdc_ images/Session1Handout.pdf** (accessed 15 August 2011)

Sustainable Development Commission (2008) *Health, Place and Nature. How outdoor environments influence health and well-being: a knowledge base*. Available at **www.sd-commission.org.uk/publications/downloads/ Outdoor_environments_and_health.pdf** (accessed 15 August 2011)

Sutton, R. (1999) The *Policy Process, London, Working Paper 118*. London: Overseas Development Institute

Swann, C. and Morgan, M. (2002) *Social Capital: insights from qualitative research*. London: Health Development Agency

Swinton, J. (2001) *Spirituality and Mental Health Care: rediscovering a forgotten dimension*. United Kingdom: Jessica Kingsley Publishers

Szabo, A. (2000) 'Physical activity and psychological dysfunction' (pp. 130–53), in Biddle, S.J.H., Fox, K.R. and Boutcher, S.H. (eds) *Physical Activity and Psychological Well-being*. London: Routledge

Taniguchi, Y., Yoshioka, N., Nakata, K., Nishizawa, T., Inagawa, H., Kohchi, C. and Soma, G. (2009) 'Mechanism for maintaining homeostasis in the immune system of the intestine'. *Anticancer Research*, 29(11): 4855–60

Taylor, A.H. (2000) 'Physical activity, anxiety, and stress: a review' (pp. 10–45), in Biddle, S.J.H., Fox, K.R. and Boutcher, S.H. (eds) *Physical Activity and Psychological Well-being*. London: Routledge

Terracciano, A. (2005) 'National character does not reflect mean personality traits levels in 49 cultures'. *Science*, 310(5745): 96–100

Tesh, S.N. (1988) *Hidden Arguments: political ideology and disease prevention policy*. New Brunswick: Rutgers University Press

Thaler, R.H. and Sunstein, C.R. (2009) *Nudge: improving decisions about health, wealth, and happiness*. London: Penguin Books

Tideswell, G. and Shutler, K. (2009) *Leading Transformational Change*. Available at **www.hefce.ac.uk/lgm/build/event/transcripts/gtks.asp** (accessed 15 August 2011)

Times Higher Education (2010) 'Get happy, and get on with it'. Available at **www.timeshighereducation.co.uk/story.asp?storycode=410055** (accessed 15 August 2011)

Tones, K. and Tilford, S. (1994) *Health Education: effectiveness, efficiency and equity* (2nd Ed). Cheltenham: Nelson Thornes Ltd

Toobert, D.J., Glasgow, R.E., Strycker, L.A., Barrera, M. Jr., Radcliffe, J.L., Wander, R.C. and Bagdade, J.D. (2003) 'Biologic and quality-of-life outcomes from the Mediterranean Lifestyle Program: a randomized clinical trial'. *Diabetes Care*, 26(8): 2288–93

Townsend, P. and Davidson, N. (1982) *Inequalities in Health: The Black Report*. Harmondsworth: Penguin

Traynor, I. (2009) *Day of the Lentil Burghers: Ghent goes veggie to lose weight and save planet*. Available at **www.guardian.co.uk/environment/2009/may/13/ghent-belgium-vegetarian-day** (accessed 15 August 2011)

Trewin, D. (2001) *Measuring Wellbeing Frameworks for Australian Social Statistics*. Canberra: Australian Bureau of Social Statistics

Trumble, S. (2010) Editorial: 'Fight or Flight'. *The Clinical Teacher*, 7(3): 151–2

Tudor-Locke, C.E., Myers, A.M., Bell, R.C., Harris, S.B. and Rodger, N.W. (2002) 'Preliminary outcome evaluation of the First Step Program: a daily physical activity intervention for individuals with type 2 diabetes'. *Patient Education and Counselling*, 47(1): 23–8

Tudor-Locke, C., Bell, R.C., Myers, A.M., Harris, S.B., Ecclestone, N.A., Lauzon, N. and Rodger, N.W. (2004) 'Controlled outcome evaluation of the First Step Program: a daily physical activity intervention for individuals with type II diabetes'. *International Journal of Obesity and Related Metabolic Disorders*, 28(1): 113–19

Tuomilehto, J., Lindstrom, J., Eriksson, J.G., Valle, T.T., Hamalainen, H., Ilanne-Parikka, P., Keinanen-Kiukaanniemi, S., Laakso, M., Louheranta, A., Rastas, M., Salminen, V. and Uusitupa, M. (2001) 'Prevention of type 2 diabetes mellitus by changes in lifestyle among subjects with impaired glucose tolerance'. *N England Journal of Medicine*, 344: 1343–50

Uchida, Y. and Kitayama, S. (2009) 'Happiness and unhappiness in east and west: themes and variations'. *Emotion*, 9: 441–56

UK Government Office for Science. (2007) *Foresight Report: Tackling obesities: future choices* (2nd Ed). Department of Innovation, Universities and Skills

UK National Ecosystem Assessment (2010a) *Progress and Steps Towards Delivery*. UNEP-WCMC, Cambridge. Available at **http://uknea.unep-wcmc.org/LinkClick.aspx?fileticket=cSqQ0kOfGJA%3d&tabid=105** (accessed 15 August 2011)

UK National Ecosystem Assessment (2010b) *'Draft Synthesis of Current Status and Recent Trends'*. Available at **http://uknea.unep-wcmc.org/LinkClick.aspx?fileticket=UIQr0mgTWWU%3d&tabid=82** (accessed 15 August 2011)

United Nations (UN) (2010) *The Millennium Development Goals Report*. New York: United Nations Department of Economic and Social Affairs

United Nations Children's Fund (UNICEF) (2007) *Child Poverty in Perspective: an overview of child welfare in rich countries – a comprehensive assessment of the lives and well-being of children and adolescents in the economically advanced nations*. New York: UNICEF

United Nations Development Programme (UNDP) (2002) *Handbook on Monitoring and Evaluating for Results*. New York: Evaluation Office

United Nations Development Programme (UNDP) (2010) *Human Development Reports*. Available at **http://hdr.undp.org/en/statistics** (accessed 15 August 2011)

US Department of Health and Human Services (1996) *Physical Activity and Health: a report of the Surgeon General*. Atlanta, GA.: US Department of Health and Human Services, Centers for Disease Control and Prevention, National Center for Chronic Disease Prevention and Health Promotion

US Physical Activity Guidelines Advisory Committee (2008) *Physical Activity Guidelines Advisory Committee Report, 2008*. Washington, DC: US Department of Health and Human Services

Üstün, B. and Jakob, R. (2005) 'Calling a spade a spade: meaningful definitions of health conditions'. *Bull WHO* 2005 (83): 802

Van der Borght, K., Havekes, R., Bos, T., Eggen, B.J.L. and Van der Zee, E.A. (2007) 'Exercise improves memory acquisition and retrieval in the Y-maze task: relationship with hippocampal neurogenesis'. *Behavioural Neuroscience*, 121(2): 324–34

Van de Weyer, C. (2005) *Changing Diets, Changing Minds: how food affects mental health and behaviour*. Available at www.sustainweb.org/foodandmentalhealth/publications_and_research/ (accessed 15 August 2011)

Von Euler, C. and Soderberg, V. (1957) 'The influence of hypothalamic thermoceptive structures on the electroencephalogram and gamma motor activity'. *Electroencephalography and Clinical Neurophysiology*, 9: 391–408

Voydanoff, P. (2007) *Work, Family, and Community: exploring interconnections*. New Jersey: Lawrence Erlbaum Associates. In Wollny *et al.* (2010)

Walt, G. (1994) *Health Policy: an introduction to process and power*. London: ZED Books

Wang, G.J., Volkow, N.D. and Fowler, J.S. (2002) 'The role of dopamine in motivation for food in humans: implications for obesity'. *BioTechniques: The International Journal of Life Sciences Methods*, 6(5): 601–9

Wanless, D. (2004) *Securing Good Health in the Whole Population*. London: Department of Health

Ware, B. (2009) *Regrets of the Dying*. Available at **www.inspirationandchai.com/Regrets-of-the-Dying.html** (accessed 15 August 2011)

Warnick, B. (2009) 'Dilemma of autonomy and happiness: Harry Brighouse on subjective wellbeing and education'. *Theory and Research in Education*, 7(1): 89–111

Warr, P. (1999) 'The measurement of well-being and other aspects of mental health'. *Journal of Occupational Psychology*, 3: 193–210

Waterman, A. (1993) 'Two conceptions of happiness: Contrasts of personal expressiveness (eudemonia) and hedonic enjoyment'. *Journal of Personality and Social Psychology*, 64: 678–91

Weed, D.L. (1995) 'Epidemiology, the humanities and public health'. *American Journal of Public Health*, 86(7): 914-18

Weiss, A., Bates, C.T. and Luciano, M. (2008) 'Happiness is a personal(ity) thing: the genetics of personality and well-being in a representative sample'. *Psychological Science*. 19(3): 205–10

Welsh Office (2009) *Power to Promote or Improve Economic, Social or Environmental Well-being: guidance to Welsh local authorities*. Cardiff: Welsh Office

Westerman, J. and Exton, S.M. (1999) 'Functional anatomy of the immune system' (Chapter 1, pp. 1–34), in Schedlowski, M. and Tewes, U. (eds) *Psychoneuroimmunology: an interdisciplinary introduction*. London: Plenum Publishers

Weston, P. and Hughes, J. (1999) 'Family Form – Family Wellbeing'. *Family Matters*, 53 (Winter): 14–20

White, J. (2007) 'Wellbeing and education: issues of culture and authority'. *Journal of Philosophy of Education*, 41(1): 17–28

Wilkinson, K.P. (1991) *The Community in Rural America*. Westport, CT: Greenwood Press

Wilkinson, R. (2000) *Mind the Gap: hierarchies, health and human evolution*. London: Weidenfeld & Nicolson

Wilkinson, R. (2007) *The Impact of Inequality: how to make sick societies healthier*. London: Routledge

Wilkinson, R. and Marmot, M. (2003) *Social Determinants of Health: the solid facts* (2nd Ed). Copenhagen: WHO

Williams, K. and Green, S. (2001) *Literature Review of Public Space and Local Environments for the Cross Cutting Review: Final Report*. Oxford: Oxford Brookes University

Wilson Committee (1963) *Final Report of the Committee on the Problem of Noise*. London: HM Stationery Office

Witek-Janusek, L., Albuquerque, K., Chroniak, K.R., Chronia, C., Durazo, R. and Mathews, H.R. (2008) 'Effect of mindfulness based stress reduction on immune function, quality of life and coping in women newly diagnosed with early stage breast cancer'. *Brain, Behaviour, and Immunity*, 22(6): 969–81

Wolinsky, F.D. (1988) *The Sociology of Health: principles, practitioners and issues* (2nd Ed). California: Wadsworth Publishing Company

Wolkowitz, O.M., Epel, E.S., Reus, V.I. and Mellon, S.H. (2010) 'Depression gets old fast: do stress and depression accelerate cell aging?' *Depression Anxiety*, 27(4): 327–38

Wollny, I., Apps, J. and Henricson, C. (2010) *Can Government Measure Family Wellbeing? A literature review*. London: Family & Parenting Institute

Woodhill, J. (2005) 'M & E as learning; rethinking the dominant paradigm', in de Graaff, J., Cameron, J., Sombatpanit, S., Pieri, C. and Woodhill, J. (2007) *Monitoring and Evaluation of Soil Conservation and Watershed Development Projects*. United States: Science Publishers

World Health Organization (WHO) (1946) *Constitution*. Geneva: WHO

World Health Organization (1948) *Preamble to the Constitution of the World Health Organization as adopted by the International Health Conference, New York, 19–22 June, 1946; signed on 22 July 1946 by the representatives of 61 States (Official Records of the World Health Organization, no. 2, p. 100) and entered into force on 7 April 1948*. Available at www.who.int/about/definition/en/print.html (accessed 15 August 2011)

World Health Organization (1981) *Global Strategy for Health for all by the year 2000*. Available at http://whqlibdoc.who.int/publications/9241800038.pdf (accessed 15 August 2011)

World Health Organization (WHO) (1984) *Health Promotion Glossary*. Geneva: WHO

World Health Organization (WHO) (1986) *Ottawa Charter for Health Promotion*. Geneva: WHO

World Health Organization (WHO) (1989) *European Charter on Environment and Health.* Available at **www.euro.who.int/__data/assets/ pdf_file/0019/114085/ICP_RUD_113.pdf** (accessed 15 August 2011)

World Health Organization (2000) *The World Health Report 2000 – Health systems: Improving performance.* Geneva: WHO

World Health Organization (WHO) (2001) *Mental Health: Strengthening mental health problems. WHO Fact Sheet 220.* Geneva: WHO

World Health Organization (WHO) (2005) *Ecosystems and Human Well-being. Health synthesis.* Available at **www.who.int/globalchange/ ecosystems/ecosys.pdf** (accessed 15 August 2011)

World Health Organization (2007) *Prevalence of Excess Body Weight and Obesity in Children and Adolescents. Fact Sheet 2.3 ENHIS.* Copenhagen: WHO

World Health Organization (WHO) (2008) *Global Burden of Disease Report.* Available at **www.who.int/healthinfo/global_burden_disease/estimates_ country/en/index.html** (accessed 15 August 2011)

World Health Organization (2009) *Public Health Campaigns: getting the message across* (Mul edition, 27 July 2009)

Wright-Mills, C. (1962) *The Power Elite.* New York: Oxford University Press

Youngstedt, S.D., O'Connor, P.J. and Dishman, R.K. (1997) 'The effects of acute exercise on sleep: a quantitative synthesis'. *Sleep,* 20(3): 203–14

Zanuso, S., Balducci, S. and Jiménez, A. (2009) 'Physical activity, a key factor to quality of life in type 2 diabetic patients'. *Diabetes/Metabolism Research & Reviews,* 25: 24–8

Index